DATE DUE

APR 1 9 1992	FEB 16 1996
OCT 3 0 1992	APR - 1 1996
NOV 1 6 1992	
FEB 1 0 1993	NOV 1 9 1996
APR 5 1993	JAN 3 1 1997
APR 2 6 1993	FEB 1 9 1997
JUN 1 1 1993	JUN 1 9 1998
SEP 2 9 1993	NOV 1 5 1998
OCT 2 3 1993	
NOV 1 0 1993	AUG 1 5 1999
DEC - 2 1993	FEB 0 4 2000
DEC 1 6 1993	APR 2 1 2001
	NOV 6 2001
FEB 1 9 1994	NOV 1 9 2002
MAR - 7 1994	
MAR 1 4 1994	
OCT - 1 1994	
JAN 2 5 1995	
NOV 2 4 1995	

BRODART, INC.   Cat. No. 23-221

PAIN

GENERAL EDITORS

Dale C. Garell, M.D.
Medical Director, California Children Services, Department of Health Services,
  County of Los Angeles
Associate Dean for Curriculum; Clinical Professor, Department of Pediatrics &
  Family Medicine, University of Southern California School of Medicine
Former President, Society for Adolescent Medicine

Solomon H. Snyder, M.D.
Distinguished Service Professor of Neuroscience, Pharmacology, and Psychiatry,
  Johns Hopkins University School of Medicine
Former President, Society for Neuroscience
Albert Lasker Award in Medical Research, 1978

CONSULTING EDITORS

Robert W. Blum, M.D., Ph.D.
Professor and Director, Division of General Pediatrics and Adolescent Health,
  University of Minnesota

Charles E. Irwin, Jr., M.D.
Professor of Pediatrics; Director, Division of Adolescent Medicine, University of
  California, San Francisco

Lloyd J. Kolbe, Ph.D.
Director of the Division of Adolescent and School Health, Center for Chronic
  Disease Prevention and Health Promotion, Centers for Disease Control

Jordan J. Popkin
Director, Division of Federal Employee Occupational Health, U.S. Public Health
  Service Region I

Joseph L. Rauh, M.D.
Professor of Pediatrics and Medicine, Adolescent Medicine, Children's Hospital
  Medical Center, Cincinnati
Former President, Society for Adolescent Medicine

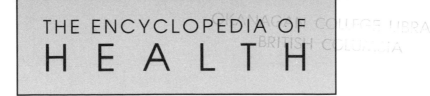

THE ENCYCLOPEDIA OF
H E A L T H

MEDICAL DISORDERS
AND THEIR TREATMENT

Dale C. Garell, M.D. • General Editor

PAIN

Mary Kittredge

Introduction by C. Everett Koop, M.D., Sc.D.

former Surgeon General, U. S. Public Health Service

CHELSEA HOUSE PUBLISHERS

New York • Philadelphia

The goal of the ENCYCLOPEDIA OF HEALTH *is to provide general information in the ever-changing areas of physiology, psychology, and related medical issues. The titles in this series are not intended to take the place of the professional advice of a physician or other health care professional.*

CHELSEA HOUSE PUBLISHERS
EDITOR-IN-CHIEF   Remmel Nunn
MANAGING EDITOR   Karyn Gullen Browne
COPY CHIEF   Mark Rifkin
PICTURE EDITOR   Adrian G. Allen
ART DIRECTOR   Maria Epes
ASSISTANT ART DIRECTOR   Noreen Romano
MANUFACTURING MANAGER   Gerald Levine
SYSTEMS MANAGER   Lindsey Ottman
PRODUCTION MANAGER   Joseph Romano
PRODUCTION COORDINATOR   Marie Claire Cebrián

The Encyclopedia of Health
SENIOR EDITOR   Brian Feinberg

Staff for PAIN
ASSOCIATE EDITOR   LaVonne Carlson-Finnerty
SENIOR COPY EDITOR   Laurie Kahn
EDITORIAL ASSISTANTS   Tamar Levovitz, Victoria Davidovsky
PICTURE RESEARCHER   Sandy Jones
DESIGNER   Robert Yaffe

First Printing
1   3   5   7   9   8   6   4   2

Library of Congress Cataloging-in-Publication Data

Kittredge, Mary.
   Pain/by Mary Kittredge; introduction by C. Everett Koop.
      p.   cm.—(The Encyclopedia of health. Medical disorders and their treatment)
   Includes bibliographical references and index.
   Summary: Discusses the nature of pain, how it manifests itself in the human body, and the medical breakthroughs in the area of pain relief.
   ISBN 0-7910-0072-9
         0-7910-0499-6 (pbk.)
   1. Pain—Juvenile literature. [1. Pain.] I. Title. II. Series.   91-3739
RB127.K45 1991   CIP
616'.0472—dc20   AC

CONTENTS

THE ENCYCLOPEDIA OF HEALTH

THE HEALTHY BODY

The Circulatory System
Dental Health
The Digestive System
The Endocrine System
Exercise
Genetics & Heredity
The Human Body: An Overview
Hygiene
The Immune System
Memory & Learning
The Musculoskeletal System
The Nervous System
Nutrition
The Reproductive System
The Respiratory System
The Senses
Sleep
Speech & Hearing
Sports Medicine
Vision
Vitamins & Minerals

THE LIFE CYCLE

Adolescence
Adulthood
Aging
Childhood
Death & Dying
The Family
Friendship & Love
Pregnancy & Birth

MEDICAL ISSUES

Careers in Health Care
Environmental Health
Folk Medicine
Health Care Delivery
Holistic Medicine
Medical Ethics
Medical Fakes & Frauds
Medical Technology
Medicine & the Law
Occupational Health
Public Health

PSYCHOLOGICAL DISORDERS AND THEIR TREATMENT

Anxiety & Phobias
Child Abuse
Compulsive Behavior
Delinquency & Criminal Behavior
Depression
Diagnosing & Treating Mental Illness
Eating Habits & Disorders
Learning Disabilities
Mental Retardation
Personality Disorders
Schizophrenia
Stress Management
Suicide

MEDICAL DISORDERS AND THEIR TREATMENT

AIDS
Allergies
Alzheimer's Disease
Arthritis
Birth Defects
Cancer
The Common Cold
Diabetes
Emergency Medicine
Gynecological Disorders
Headaches
The Hospital
Kidney Disorders
Medical Diagnosis
The Mind-Body Connection
Mononucleosis and Other Infectious Diseases
Nuclear Medicine
Organ Transplants
Pain
Physical Handicaps
Poisons & Toxins
Prescription & OTC Drugs
Sexually Transmitted Diseases
Skin Disorders
Stroke & Heart Disease
Substance Abuse
Tropical Medicine

PREVENTION
AND
EDUCATION:
THE KEYS
TO GOOD HEALTH

C. Everett Koop, M.D., Sc.D.
former Surgeon General,
U.S. Public Health Service

The issue of health education has received particular attention in recent years because of the presence of AIDS in the news. But our response to this particular tragedy points up a number of broader issues that doctors, public health officials, educators, and the public face. In particular, it points up the necessity for sound health education for citizens of all ages.

Over the past 25 years this country has been able to bring about dramatic declines in the death rates for heart disease, stroke, accidents, and for people under the age of 45, cancer. Today, Americans generally eat better and take better care of themselves than ever before. Thus, with the help of modern science and technology, they have a better chance of surviving serious—even catastrophic—illnesses. That's the good news.

But, like every phonograph record, there's a flip side, and one with special significance for young adults. According to a report issued in 1979 by Dr. Julius Richmond, my predecessor as Surgeon General, Americans aged 15 to 24 had a higher death rate in 1979 than they did 20 years earlier. The causes: violent death and injury, alcohol and drug abuse, unwanted pregnancies, and sexually transmitted diseases. Adolescents are particularly vulnerable because they are beginning to explore their own sexuality and perhaps to experiment with drugs. The need for educating young people is critical, and the price of neglect is high.

Yet even for the population as a whole, our health is still far from what it could be. Why? A 1974 Canadian government report attributed all death and disease to four broad elements: inadequacies in the health care system, behavioral factors or unhealthy life-styles, environmental hazards, and human biological factors.

7

To be sure, there are diseases that are still beyond the control of even our advanced medical knowledge and techniques. And despite yearnings that are as old as the human race itself, there is no "fountain of youth" to ward off aging and death. Still, there is a solution to many of the problems that undermine sound health. In a word, that solution is prevention. Prevention, which includes health promotion and education, saves lives, improves the quality of life, and in the long run, saves money.

In the United States, organized public health activities and preventive medicine have a long history. Important milestones in this country or foreign breakthroughs adopted in the United States include the improvement of sanitary procedures and the development of pasteurized milk in the late 19th century and the introduction in the mid-20th century of effective vaccines against polio, measles, German measles, mumps, and other once-rampant diseases. Internationally, organized public health efforts began on a wide-scale basis with the International Sanitary Conference of 1851, to which 12 nations sent representatives. The World Health Organization, founded in 1948, continues these efforts under the aegis of the United Nations, with particular emphasis on combating communicable diseases and the training of health care workers.

Despite these accomplishments, much remains to be done in the field of prevention. For too long, we have had a medical care system that is science- and technology-based, focused, essentially, on illness and mortality. It is now patently obvious that both the social and the economic costs of such a system are becoming insupportable.

Implementing prevention—and its corollaries, health education and promotion—is the job of several groups of people.

First, the medical and scientific professions need to continue basic scientific research, and here we are making considerable progress. But increased concern with prevention will also have a decided impact on how primary care doctors practice medicine. With a shift to health-based rather than morbidity-based medicine, the role of the "new physician" will include a healthy dose of patient education.

Second, practitioners of the social and behavioral sciences—psychologists, economists, city planners—along with lawyers, business leaders, and government officials—must solve the practical and ethical dilemmas confronting us: poverty, crime, civil rights, literacy, education, employment, housing, sanitation, environmental protection, health care delivery systems, and so forth. All of these issues affect public health.

Third is the public at large. We'll consider that very important group in a moment.

Fourth, and the linchpin in this effort, is the public health profession—doctors, epidemiologists, teachers—who must harness the professional expertise of the first two groups and the common sense and cooperation of the third, the public. They must define the problems statistically and qualitatively and then help us set priorities for finding the solutions.

To a very large extent, improving those statistics is the responsibility of every individual. So let's consider more specifically what the role of the individual should be and why health education is so important to that role. First, and most obvious, individuals can protect themselves from illness and injury and thus minimize their need for professional medical care. They can eat nutritious food; get adequate exercise; avoid tobacco, alcohol, and drugs; and take prudent steps to avoid accidents. The proverbial "apple a day keeps the doctor away" is not so far from the truth, after all.

Second, individuals should actively participate in their own medical care. They should schedule regular medical and dental checkups. Should they develop an illness or injury, they should know when to treat themselves and when to seek professional help. To gain the maximum benefit from any medical treatment that they do require, individuals must become partners in that treatment. For instance, they should understand the effects and side effects of medications. I counsel young physicians that there is no such thing as too much information when talking with patients. But the corollary is the patient must know enough about the nuts and bolts of the healing process to understand what the doctor is telling him or her. That is at least partially the patient's responsibility.

Education is equally necessary for us to understand the ethical and public policy issues in health care today. Sometimes individuals will encounter these issues in making decisions about their own treatment or that of family members. Other citizens may encounter them as jurors in medical malpractice cases. But we all become involved, indirectly, when we elect our public officials, from school board members to the president. Should surrogate parenting be legal? To what extent is drug testing desirable, legal, or necessary? Should there be public funding for family planning, hospitals, various types of medical research, and other medical care for the indigent? How should we allocate scant technological resources, such as kidney dialysis and organ transplants? What is the proper role of government in protecting the rights of patients?

What are the broad goals of public health in the United States today? In 1980, the Public Health Service issued a report aptly entitled *Promoting Health—Preventing Disease: Objectives for the Nation*. This report expressed its goals in terms of mortality and in terms of intermediate goals in education and health improvement. It identified 15 major concerns: controlling high blood pressure; improving family planning; improving pregnancy care and infant health; increasing the rate of immunization; controlling sexually transmitted diseases; controlling the presence of toxic agents and radiation in the environment; improving occupational safety and health; preventing accidents; promoting water fluoridation and dental health; controlling infectious diseases; decreasing smoking; decreasing alcohol and drug abuse; improving nutrition; promoting physical fitness and exercise; and controlling stress and violent behavior.

For healthy adolescents and young adults (ages 15 to 24), the specific goal was a 20% reduction in deaths, with a special focus on motor vehicle injuries and alcohol and drug abuse. For adults (ages 25 to 64), the aim was 25% fewer deaths, with a concentration on heart attacks, strokes, and cancers.

Smoking is perhaps the best example of how individual behavior can have a direct impact on health. Today, cigarette smoking is recognized as the single most important preventable cause of death in our society. It is responsible for more cancers and more cancer deaths than any other known agent; is a prime risk factor for heart and blood vessel disease, chronic bronchitis, and emphysema; and is a frequent cause of complications in pregnancies and of babies born prematurely, underweight, or with potentially fatal respiratory and cardiovascular problems.

Since the release of the Surgeon General's first report on smoking in 1964, the proportion of adult smokers has declined substantially, from 43% in 1965 to 30.5% in 1985. Since 1965, 37 million people have quit smoking. Although there is still much work to be done if we are to become a "smoke-free society," it is heartening to note that public health and public education efforts—such as warnings on cigarette packages and bans on broadcast advertising—have already had significant effects.

In 1835, Alexis de Tocqueville, a French visitor to America, wrote, "In America the passion for physical well-being is general." Today, as then, health and fitness are front-page items. But with the greater scientific and technological resources now available to us, we are in a far stronger position to make good health care available to everyone. And with the greater technological threats to us as we approach the 21st century, the need to do so is more urgent than ever before. Comprehensive information about basic biology, preventive medicine, medical and surgical treatments, and related ethical and public policy issues can help you arm yourself with the knowledge you need to be healthy throughout your life.

FOREWORD

Dale C. Garell, M.D.

Advances in our understanding of health and disease during the 20th century have been truly remarkable. Indeed, it could be argued that modern health care is one of the greatest accomplishments in all of human history. In the early 20th century, improvements in sanitation, water treatment, and sewage disposal reduced death rates and increased longevity. Previously untreatable illnesses can now be managed with antibiotics, immunizations, and modern surgical techniques. Discoveries in the fields of immunology, genetic diagnosis, and organ transplantation are revolutionizing the prevention and treatment of disease. Modern medicine is even making inroads against cancer and heart disease, two of the leading causes of death in the United States.

Although there is much to be proud of, medicine continues to face enormous challenges. Science has vanquished diseases such as smallpox and polio, but new killers, most notably AIDS, confront us. Moreover, we now victimize ourselves with what some have called "diseases of choice," or those brought on by drug and alcohol abuse, bad eating habits, and mismanagement of the stresses and strains of contemporary life. The very technology that is doing so much to prolong life has brought with it previously unimaginable ethical dilemmas related to issues of death and dying. The rising cost of health care is a matter of central concern to us all. And violence in the form of automobile accidents, homicide, and suicide remains the major killer of young adults.

In the past, most people were content to leave health care and medical treatment in the hands of professionals. But since the 1960s, the consumer of medical care—that is, the patient—has assumed an increasingly central role in the management of his or her own health. There has also been a new emphasis placed on prevention: People are recognizing that their own actions can help prevent many of the conditions that have caused death and disease in the past. This accounts for the growing commitment to good nutrition and regular exercise, for the increasing number of people who are choosing not to smoke, and for a new moderation in people's drinking habits.

People want to know more about themselves and their own health. They are curious about their body: its anatomy, physiology, and bio-chemistry. They want to keep up with rapidly evolving medical tech-nologies and procedures. They are willing to educate themselves about common disorders and diseases so that they can be full partners in their own health care.

THE ENCYCLOPEDIA OF HEALTH is designed to provide the basic knowledge that readers will need if they are to take significant respon-sibility for their own health. It is also meant to serve as a frame of reference for further study and exploration. The encyclopedia is divided into five subsections: The Healthy Body; The Life Cycle; Medical Disorders & Their Treatment; Psychological Disorders & Their Treatment; and Medi-cal Issues. For each topic covered by the encyclopedia, we present the essential facts about the relevant biology; the symptoms, diagnosis, and treatment of common diseases and disorders; and ways in which you can prevent or reduce the severity of health problems when that is possible. The encyclopedia also projects what may lie ahead in the way of future treatment or prevention strategies.

The broad range of topics and issues covered in the encyclopedia reflects that human health encompasses physical, psychological, social, environmental, and spiritual well-being. Just as the mind and the body are inextricably linked, so, too, is the individual an integral part of the wider world that comprises his or her family, society, and environment. To discuss health in its broadest aspect it is necessary to explore the many ways in which it is connected to such fields as law, social science, public policy, economics, and even religion. And so, the encyclopedia is meant to be a bridge between science, medical technology, the world at large, and you. I hope that it will inspire you to pursue in greater depth particular areas of interest and that you will take advantage of the suggestions for further reading and the lists of resources and organizations that can provide additional information.

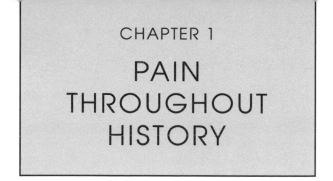

CHAPTER 1

PAIN THROUGHOUT HISTORY

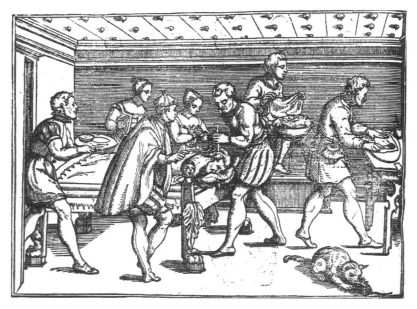

Through the ages, people have tried to ease pain in a variety of ways. This 1573 wood engraving demonstrates trephining—that is, drilling into the skull to relieve tension. A form of this surgery is still used today.

Throughout history people have searched for ways to avoid or relieve pain. As early as 6,000 years ago in the Middle East, Sumerian healers used opium to deaden pain. Ancient Greeks and Romans also used this drug derived from the poppy plant, believing that it summoned the god of sleep to relieve pain. The ancient Greek physician Hippocrates used ice and applied pressure on large blood vessels to numb pain. Healers of ancient India used hashish and a medicine made from mandrake roots to ease a variety of discomforts.

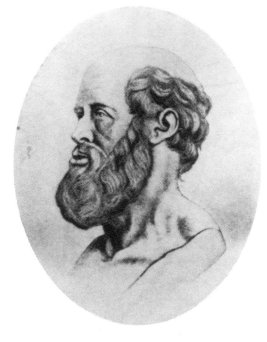

The renowned Greek physician Hippocrates (ca. 460–ca. 377 B.C.) numbed pain by placing ice on an injury or by applying pressure to a large blood vessel.

Several thousand years ago in China, the legendary healer Hua T'o had such wide knowledge of painkilling drugs and techniques, including *acupuncture* (a way of easing pain by inserting needles into specific points on the body), that he was worshiped as a god. In South America, healers used potions made from coca leaves (the source of the modern drug cocaine) to numb the pain of an early type of brain surgery called *trephining*, the opening of a patient's skull to let out evil spirits thought to cause headaches and other illnesses.

In early Christian times, pain was seen as a means of purification, a way to wash away sins and prove one's devotion. Sufferers were advised to pray for relief and to offer up their pain to God as a way to save their own soul and the souls of others. Some devout worshipers, called *flagellants*, even inflicted pain upon themselves; remnants of these groups still exist, not only among Christians but also among Hindus, Muslims, and observers of many other faiths. Suffering for spiritual reasons was part of certain early Native American religions as well. The North American Plains Indians performed a ritual sun dance wherein young men hung themselves from daggers inserted into their chests to prove their manhood and become holy warriors. In many primitive cultures, painful cuts that left scars were inflicted as badges of bravery and maturity.

THE SEARCH FOR RELIEF

For most people, deliberate endurance of suffering is secondary to the search for new and better methods of relief. After about the 9th century A.D., Persian healers grew highly skilled in these techniques. By the 10th century, the Persian physician Avicenna had written a 5-volume book of medicine, including one whole book listing all the known varieties of pain along with drugs and techniques for relieving them. Trade with Italy, and the Crusades, brought some of this knowledge to European lands, where Christian monks began to quietly practice healing arts.

Early Anesthesia

The monastery at Monte Cassino was the site of the 11th-century operation to remove kidney stones from King Henry II of Bavaria. Pope Victor II's account of this event included a suggestion that the monks had put the king to sleep by giving him vapors to inhale before the surgery. Interestingly, *general anesthesia*—breathing a sleep-producing gas to relieve the surgical pain—was not discovered by modern surgeons until the 1700s. Yet a recipe for making drug-soaked sponges

The belief that suffering is a path to spiritual purity is held by followers of religions across the globe. When taken to extremes, those devotees who actually inflict pain on themselves are referred to as flagellants, depicted in this 1721 woodcut.

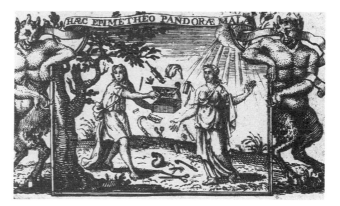

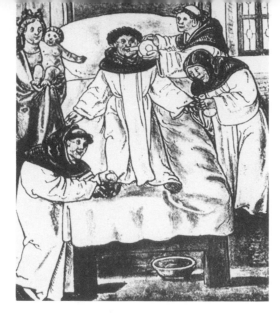

This 16th-century illustration depicts the early use of anesthetic gases for surgery. The first examples of the technique appear in the records of 11th-century monasteries, although administration of anesthesia was not generally accepted until the 19th century.

(containing opium, juice of mandrake root, and other vegetable juices) to apply to a patient's nose was discovered among the manuscripts in the monastery, showing that the Benedictines could indeed have given a primitive general anesthetic to the king. In the area of pain relief they were ahead of modern science by more than five centuries.

In the 16th century, the Swiss physician Paracelsus performed a variety of experiments with chemicals. When he mixed sulfuric acid with alcohol and tested the mixture on chickens, he found that it temporarily put them to sleep. Although other scientists knew about the substance, they had not recognized it as a painkiller. In fact, the substance was *ether*, a compound with vapors that are a safe and effective general anesthetic when inhaled. Yet ether would not be purified and used as an anesthetic for another 300 years, because the medical principles for producing and using such gases were not yet known or understood. Meanwhile, physicians explored other methods of pain relief.

Applying Pressure

By the 18th century, physicians knew that pressing on blood vessels in the neck could block blood flow to the brain and produce unconsciousness. Next, they tried pressing on nerves to block sensation—and pain—without making a patient unconscious. In 1784, English scien-

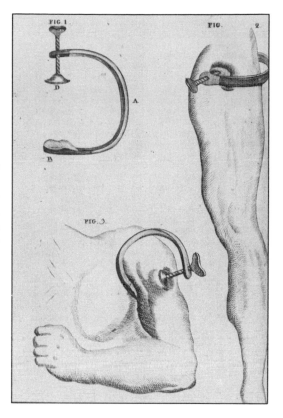

Eighteenth-century surgeons numbed the body during surgery by compressing blood vessels and blocking circulation to the nerves of the injured area.

tist James Moore invented a device that would deaden pain by *nerve blocking*. It was used by famed English surgeon John Hunter for amputating legs.

Nonphysical means of pain relief were also tried in the 18th century, particularly when the techniques of Austrian physician Franz Mesmer gained great popularity. Mesmer believed that the body contained magnetic fluids and that manipulating these fluids could cure pains and diseases. At first he used real magnets, but later said he could magnetize an ordinary stick and use it like a magic wand to draw the illness from a person's body.

Many important people, including Marie Antoinette of France, made Mesmer rich and famous. When he could not cure someone, he explained away his failure by saying that the individual did not really want to be cured. Actually, Mesmer's techniques mainly worked on people's pocketbooks, and in 1784 a commission appointed by the French government exposed him as a fraud.

However, Mesmer had taught his techniques to a French nobleman named de Puygesur, who added hand motions and strong suggestions to the method. He used his adaptation of the method, called *mesmerism*, on a young man and unexpectedly put him into a trance. He had, without knowing it, invented *hypnotism*, a state resembling sleep that is induced by a person whose suggestions are easily accepted by a subject.

By the early 19th century, hypnotism was being used to prevent pain during surgery in France, England, Austria, and the United States. An English surgeon in India, James Esdaile, performed 600 painless operations on patients whom he had put into a hypnotic trance. However, the physical sciences such as chemistry, anatomy (the study of the body's construction), and physiology (the study of how the body's structures work) were making great strides at the same time, which caused hypnotism to lose its influence as the standard way of relieving pain.

GENERAL ANESTHETIC GASES

Meanwhile, other discoveries were made in the fight against pain. Scientists had begun to combine bits of knowledge they had learned about the body in the 17th century: The English physician William Harvey found that blood circulates around the body, and the English chemist Robert Boyle discovered that breathing moves oxygen into the blood. Taken together, the two findings suggested that other substances might also be inhaled and sent through the body by way of the

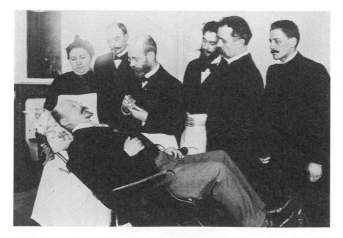

French physicians observe a colleague hypnotizing a patient; although it was primarily used to treat victims of mental disorders in 18th-century Europe, hypnotism was not developed for surgical purposes until the following century.

bloodstream—which in turn suggested that gases that cause unconsciousness could be used to relieve the pain of surgery. Thus, the usefulness of anesthetic gases, as well as reliable ways of administering them, were finally developed 300 years after the discovery of ether. Because scientists were better able to explain anesthetic gases and their effects on the body than the mysterious techniques and results of hypnotism, they were inclined to accept and use the gases.

In 1844, a Connecticut dentist named Horace Wells used ether to extract a patient's tooth without pain. In 1846, ether was used during surgery for a neck tumor. By the 1850s, a similar gas called *chloroform* was used to stop pain in childbirth and many kinds of major and minor surgery. Another gas, *nitrous oxide*, was also found to be a useful general anesthetic. In the few years that followed, the techniques of administering the gases safely and mixing them with oxygen were refined, so that by the early 20th century, the use of general anesthetics was commonplace. Painless surgery was no longer the miraculous exception, but the rule, and helped lead to an increase in the types of lifesaving surgery that could be performed.

Local Anesthetics

Over the same period, *local anesthetics*, drugs that kill pain without rendering the patient unconscious, were also more fully investigated. The Viennese surgeon Carl Koller introduced the use of cocaine for eye surgery in 1884. Later, American surgeon William Halsted injected the drug into nerves to produce numbness in a specific part of the body. By 1898, German surgeon August Bier had learned that injecting cocaine into the spinal cord could produce temporary numbness in the entire lower body. However, the dangerous side effects of cocaine, especially its tendency to increase the heart rate, led to the substitution of other drugs such as *lidocaine* and *novocaine*.

The year 1903 brought a further advance against pain: the development of the *barbiturate* class of drugs. Barbiturates are addictive drugs, such as *phenobarbital*, that produce calmness or sleep. Injecting barbiturates into the bloodstream was an effective way of easing anxiety before and after surgery.

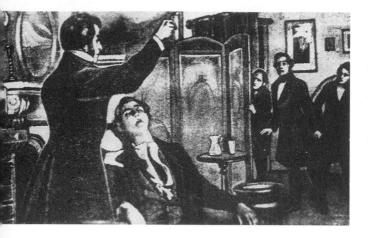

"A new era in tooth pulling," was declared by dentist Horace Wells in 1844, when he first used gas as a general anesthetic for extracting wisdom teeth.

Throughout the 20th century, modern chemistry has produced painkilling anesthetics that are much improved over the first substances used to produce unconsciousness or deaden pain. These include synthetic narcotics such as *Dilaudid*, *meperidine*, and *methadone*; general anesthetics such as *halothane*; and local anesthetics safe enough to be used even without a prescription, such as *benzocaine*. (Except for the nonprescription local anesthetics, these drugs have serious side effects and should only be given by a physician.)

Oral Analgesics

Also during the 20th century, another class of painkillers was refined, the *oral analgesics*. Taken by mouth, these drugs relieve minor aches and pains such as headaches, toothaches, and muscle aches. Although they can often be purchased without a prescription, they are drugs and can produce harmful side effects. Therefore, they should be taken with care, and only according to directions.

The first of these drugs, *aspirin*, was known in primitive form by American Indians, who used a potion made from the bark of willow trees to relieve pain. The bark was studied in the early 20th century by workers at the Bayer Company in Germany, who found the active ingredient was *acetylsalicylic acid*. The purified substance became the basis of brand name analgesics that are still in use today, including Bromo-Seltzer and Bayer aspirin. But no one knew how aspirin worked until the latter half of the century, when Swedish scientists Sune

Bergstrom, Bengt Samuelsson, and colleague Sir John Vane found that it interferes with the body's production of *prostaglandin*, a potent pain-producing substance.

Acetaminophen, sold under names such as Tylenol and Datril, is an aspirinlike synthetic drug with much the same effect as aspirin. It is especially useful as an aspirin substitute for individuals under age 16, because aspirin has been linked to an ailment in young people called *Reye's syndrome*. This is a sometimes fatal complication of flu, chicken pox, and other viral illnesses. Hence, the American Academy of Pediatrics recommends that children and young adults use acetaminophen rather than aspirin for relief of aches and fever during such illnesses.

Among the newest of the oral analgesics is the drug *ibuprofen*, first sold as a prescription drug under the brand name Motrin. Developed for the relief of joint inflammation (such as arthritis) and severe menstrual cramps, it is now available without prescription under brand names such as Nuprin and Advil. Its chemical formula is completely different from that of aspirin, so it is especially recommended for people who are allergic to aspirin.

RESEARCH

Research into the basic causes and mechanisms of pain is another essential aspect of the search for better pain relief. Study of the nervous system has produced a number of ideas on how pain occurs and how it is transmitted to and perceived by the brain. The scientific field of molecular biology—the study of how *molecules* (the smallest possible

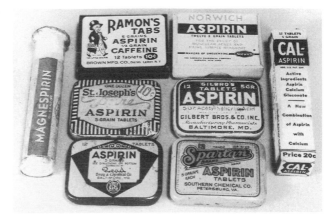

Today's most popular painkiller has prehistoric origins. Native Americans originally obtained its main ingredient from willow bark, yet aspirin was not put into pill form and commonly used until the 20th century.

measure of a substance) behave in living things—promises to reveal even more about how human nerve and brain cells, as well as the tiny structures within these cells, behave when pain occurs. (*Cells* are the basic building blocks of which all living matter is made.) The study of specific pains, such as headaches, is also producing information about pain's causes and cures.

Psychology, the study of the ways people perceive and understand things, is helping doctors learn more about the experience of pain, and how a patient's mind and emotions may affect it. *Pharmacology*, the study of drugs, continues the search for better medicines that relieve pain. In this area, the study of the brain's own pain-relieving substances offers hope that improved and less addictive medicines may be developed.

Experts in a wide range of sciences, from *medical engineering* (the study of medical devices) to *anesthesiology* (the medical specialty of pain relief, especially in surgery), also continue to work for a better understanding of pain and improved techniques for prevention and relief.

Finally, the care of the people who suffer pain has become a medical specialty in the latter part of the 20th century. Physicians today may refer people with severe or supposedly incurable pain to specialized clinics where experts offer a highly specialized level of help. According to Dr. Joel Saper, director of the Michigan Headache and Neurological Institute, 9 out of 10 sufferers of severe, chronic headaches can now get relief at headache clinics.

Increasingly, pain is being seen as a serious problem in itself, not just a side effect of some other ailment, and is being scrutinized by scientific organizations, such as the International Association for the Study of Pain. In addition, the monthly medical journal *Pain* provides a forum for specialists worldwide to report progress in the field. A self-help group for victims of chronic pain, the American Chronic Pain Association, offers information and support, and the International Pain Foundation is a professional organization that helps raise money for research and education. Fortunately, modern scientific insights into the workings of the human body have provided doctors with a better understanding of pain and its relief than at any other time in history.

CHAPTER 2

PLACES WHERE PAIN OCCURS

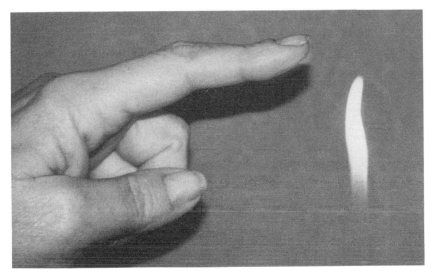

Pain is not merely a reminder that an injury has already occurred; it actually involves a complex series of reactions to warn the sufferer against previously unrecognized problems and to prevent further damage.

A fingertip touches a burning match. The heat of the flame begins searing the skin at once, but no pain is felt until lightning-fast nerve messages race from the skin to the brain, carrying damage reports. This delay occurs because the burned place does not really feel anything until the brain tells it to: The injury damages the finger, but the brain produces pain. This appears simple because the pain occurs quickly—in just a fraction of a second—and seems to affect only the injured site (the burned fingertip, for example). But pain is actually produced through a complex process, involving separate steps that occur at the site of the injury, in nerves that link the injured area with the brain, and within the brain itself.

The body uses a variety of nerve cells to perceive the many possible types of sensations. The free endings primarily gain information through the skin, and the capsule-shaped endings gather data from within the body.

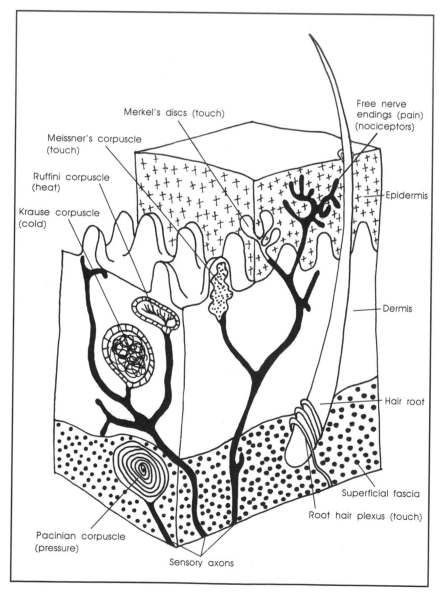

WHERE PAIN BEGINS

The first phase of pain, called *nociception*, occurs when special nerve endings react to an injury such as a burn, cut, or blow. Nerve endings

The peripheral nervous system carries messages from outlying areas of the body to the central nervous system, which uses the spinal cord to relay messages to the brain.

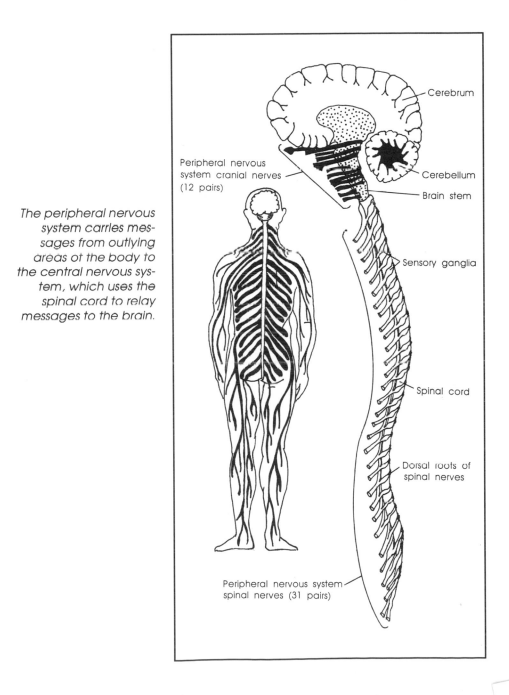

are distributed generously throughout the body; up to 1,300 of them may cover 1 square inch of skin. These nerve endings are responsible for gathering the information received through the sense of touch—sensations of heat, cold, contact, and pressure, as well as pain. Some, called *free endings*, are like tiny networks of lace; others are tiny capsule-shaped bodies. The free endings gather information mostly from outside the body, through the skin. The capsule-shaped endings are more numerous inside the body, for example, in joints, muscles, and internal organs. (The brain is an exception because none of its nerve cells are designed to gather touch or pain messages.)

Free endings are also the kind of nerve endings that react to injury by sending pain signals. Scientists are not sure whether all free endings can be pain reactors or if the body has a set especially for pain; however, any nerve ending that can sense pain is called a *nociceptor*. Some nociceptors sense sharp blows, others sense heat, and a third kind senses a variety of pressure, temperature, and chemical changes.

THE PERIPHERAL NERVOUS SYSTEM

When free endings are cut, burned, or injured in other ways, nociception occurs: The nociceptors transmit damage reports to a vast network of other nerves called the *peripheral nervous system*. The peripheral nervous system is located outside the *central nervous system* (which consists of the brain and spinal cord) and registers physical sensations. Two kinds of messages move along this network: *afferent messages*, which carry information to the brain about the outside world or about the body itself; and *efferent messages*, which deliver instructions from the brain to the body.

In order to communicate, each nerve cell in the peripheral nervous system is linked to the next by tiny branches, called *axons* and *dendrites*. Each nerve cell has many dendrites to receive messages and a single long axon to send them. Each axon in the peripheral nervous system is lined with smaller cells called *neuroglia*. These cells are coated with a fatty substance called *myelin* that insulates axons so that

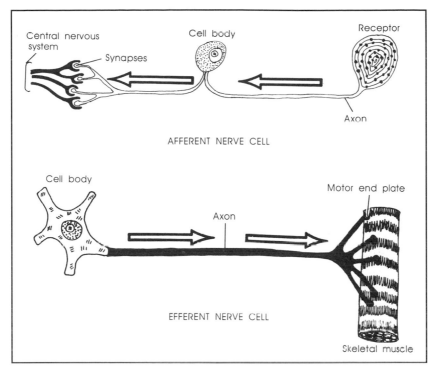

Two types of nerve cells transmit information between the body and the brain: Afferent nerves relay messages from the outside world or the body itself to the brain; efferent nerves carry instructions from the brain to the body.

they will not send misdirected messages to neighboring axons. The only part of the axon that is not covered by neuroglia is a small area near a tiny gap. This gap is called a *synapse*; it lies between the axon of one nerve cell and a dendrite of the next.

How Nerve Signals Travel

Once a pain message is received from a capsule-shaped or free ending, it moves through one peripheral nerve cell after another on its way to the brain. Before a message arrives, a typical nerve cell, called a *neuron*, contains potassium *ions*. (Ions are atoms or groups of atoms

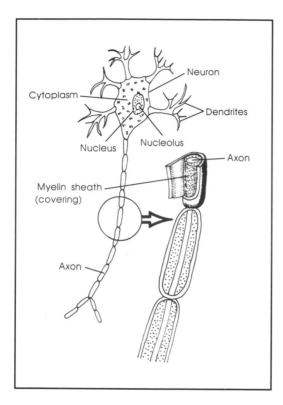

Cytoplasm

Neuron

Dendrites

Nucleus

Nucleolus

Axon

Myelin sheath (covering)

Axon

Each nerve cell has two types of message sensors: The dendrites receive an incoming message; the axon passes it to the next nerve cell.

that carry an electrical charge.) The neuron, in turn, is surrounded by fluid containing sodium ions.

To send a nerve impulse, a neuron fires a burst of chemicals called *neurotransmitters* from the end of its axon. In less than a thousandth of a second, the neurotransmitters flow across the synapse and lock onto the dendrites of the receiving neuron. In the receiving neuron, the neurotransmitters cause potassium ions to leak out and sodium ions to leak in. The receiving neuron then forces one set of ions out and takes another set of ions back in again to restore its ions to a normal state.

This flip-flop of ions moves through the neuron to the tip of the axon, which is covered by tiny bumps called *telodendrions*. The telodendrions contain tiny sacs called *synaptic vessels* that burst open to release more neurotransmitters—which jump the next synapse, enter the next neuron, and start the process all over again.

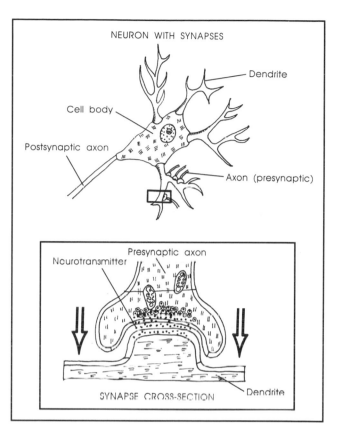

When electrical signals traveling through a nerve cell reach the end of an axon, chemicals (called neurotransmitters) are released into the gap, or synapse, leading to the next nerve cell. Upon reaching the next cell, this chemical message is transformed back into electrical impulses, and the chain reaction continues.

One of the better-understood neurotransmitters is *acetylcholine*, a chemical responsible for carrying messages from one nerve cell to the next. When the synaptic vessels release acetylcholine, it helps make the dendrites' walls permeable to the electrically charged ions that leak in and out of the dendrites of the next nerve cell. Thus, pain messages move in two ways: chemically between neurons and electrically when inside them.

Within the peripheral nervous system, messages move along two kinds of nerve fibers. Very thin ones, called *C fibers*, transmit pain signals that are felt as dull, aching, general pains. The slightly thicker *A-delta fibers* send signals for sharp pains that appear in one spot. Pain messages travel along these two kinds of fibers until they reach the spinal cord.

THE CENTRAL NERVOUS SYSTEM

The Spinal Cord

The spinal cord can be viewed as the main highway for brain-body communications. It is a ropelike structure about 18 inches long composed of nerve tissue situated inside the bones of the *spinal column.* The spinal cord runs from the base of the spine up to the brain, and branching off from it are 31 pairs of large *spinal nerves.*

A pain message traveling along a spinal nerve reaches a knoblike structure, called a *ganglion,* attached to the spinal cord. After entering the spinal cord via the ganglion, about 70% of pain messages cross to the opposite side of the cord before continuing toward the brain. Thus, a pain message from the left hand will travel up the right side of the spinal cord, and vice versa.

Within the spinal cord, pain messages move along two main routes—the *paleospinothalamic tract* and the *neospinothalamic tract.* The first means "the old (paleo) route along the spinal cord to the *thalamus*" (an area in the base of the brain). The second means "the new (neo) route along the spinal cord to the thalamus." The human

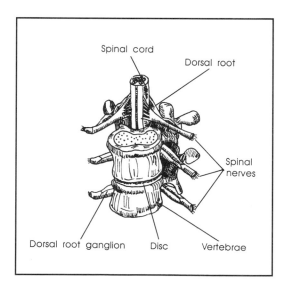

Spinal cord

Dorsal root

Spinal nerves

Dorsal root ganglion   Disc   Vertebrae

The spinal column, composed of a series of bones, nerves, and tissues, provides a central route for the body and the brain to relay messages.

body developed the paleo route earlier in its evolution: It tends to be slower, less efficient, and to send a duller, more generalized kind of pain. The neo route developed more recently: It sends faster, sharper, and easier-to-locate pain signals.

The Brain

Whichever tract they move in, pain messages eventually reach an area atop the spinal cord, near the base of the skull, called the *reticular formation*, a web of nerve cells that fans out to make contact between many brain centers. This in turn sends the pain messages to the body's central information-processing unit, the brain. There the message is received by the thalamus, which acts as a message-sorting-and-transferring station.

The thalamus instantly begins to send two kinds of messages: signals that tell the body to stop sending pain messages (once the brain has received information about the injury, no more messages about it are needed) and information about the pain message itself. This second group of signals is transmitted to the *cerebral cortex*, the thinking part of the brain that contains most of the brain's nerve cells and that actually recognizes the painful sensation. The unpleasant experience of pain, therefore, is produced not directly by the injury itself but by the cerebral cortex in response to damage reports it receives from the injury site.

At the same time it receives the pain message and produces the pain sensation, the cerebral cortex gathers and processes other information: where damage is occurring, the cause, how it can be stopped, and what can be done to prevent further damage. To obtain these answers, the cerebral cortex uses information from all of the senses. For instance, the sight of a flaming match near the skin, the sound of sizzling, and the smell of smoke, all tell the brain what is happening.

The cerebral cortex also uses information it has learned in the past. Combining memories with new information from the five senses, the cortex can determine how serious a situation is and what to do about it. Then it sends instructions to the body through the nervous system: Get the match away from the skin! Run cold water on the burn! The

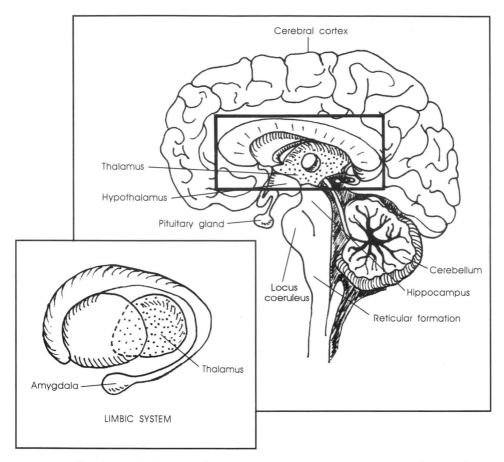

Contained within the limbic system, the cerebral cortex is the portion of the brain responsible for emotional reactions to pain; these are partially based on memories of prior experiences with pain.

cortex also stores information about the event in memory to avoid similar injuries in the future.

THE LIMBIC SYSTEM

The brain's perception of the pain process is assisted and expanded by the *limbic system*. Made up of a group of brain structures near the thalamus, the limbic system stimulates the cerebral cortex to notice certain messages with special intensity. It does so via one of its structures, called the *hippocampus*, which continually compares new messages to those that have already been received by and stored in the brain. As messages pass via the reticular formation to the cerebral cortex, the hippocampus tells the cerebral cortex to pay special attention to new or strange ones. This explains why a strange sound in a quiet house alerts people at once, and why a new pain is immediately noticed.

The limbic system also regulates the secondary effects of pain because its nerve fibers extend into many different areas of the brain. For example, it affects the hunger and pleasure centers in a part of the brain near the thalamus called the *hypothalamus*, which in turn controls many of the body's automatic functions. Pain may cause a person to lose his or her appetite when signals from the limbic system depress the hunger centers. On the other hand, sudden relief of pain may be experienced as pleasure when pain signals disappear and the pleasure center signals continue to work.

The limbic system also plays a part in the emotions people feel toward pain, such as sadness or anger. These reactions are affected by a structure in the limbic system called the *amygdala*. The amygdala not

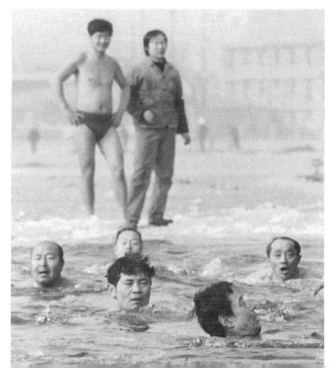

The Polar Bear Club is a worldwide organization for those who enjoy cold-water swimming. The limbic system is thought to contain the mechanisms that make diving into cold water pleasant for some people and painful for others.

only produces emotions in response to messages traveling to the cerebral cortex, it also causes the cortex to respond again to messages after they leave the amygdala. This is why pain feels worse for a person who is anxious, lonely, or sad: Unhappy emotions created in the amygdala intensify the way the cerebral cortex perceives pain messages.

In addition, the limbic system helps the cerebral cortex determine whether or not to experience a sensation as pain at all. This can be related to the circumstances surrounding the situation. Jumping into a lake of icy water, for instance, can be painful if a person has had a near-drowning experience in cold weather. But it can be pleasant if a person associates the experience with the icy bath commonly taken after a sauna by people who relish the intense sensation that results. Thus, the limbic system and the cerebral cortex can work together to turn a strong sensation to pain or to pleasure, depending in part upon the circumstances under which each individual last experienced it.

The entire process of feeling pain takes but a fraction of a second. Hardly any time at all passes between burning oneself and yelling, "Ouch!" Yet pain is the result of complex communication and a reaction involving the body, the peripheral nervous system, the spinal cord, and several different parts of the brain.

Nor is this the entire story of how pain happens. A number of the body's chemicals—at the injury site, in the peripheral nervous system, and in the brain—help to transmit and regulate pain messages and pain sensations. The next chapter looks more closely at these natural pain chemicals—what they are, where and how they are produced, and how they work to influence the production, communication, sensation, and relief of the unpleasant experience called pain.

CHAPTER 3

HOW PAIN HAPPENS

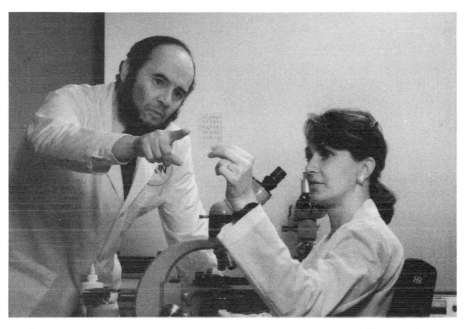

Scientists at the National Institute of Dental Research (NIDR) examine spinal cord tissue sections to learn more about neurotransmitters, thus contributing to knowledge of the body's pain pathways.

For pain to be felt, events in several widely separated structures of the nervous system take place. Nociception occurs in the pain-sensing nerve endings of the injury site. Transmission is performed by nerve fibers of the peripheral and central nervous systems. Pain messages are sent to the brain via the structure at the top of the spinal cord, the reticular formation. Perception and emotion, along with the feeling of pain itself, are produced within the brain.

But nervous system structures involved in sensing, transmitting, feeling, and reacting to pain do not by themselves create the entire pain experience. Each step of the pain process also depends on chemicals that produce, transmit, and modify pain. Created in the nervous system, these chemicals also use this system to send messages throughout the body. Without them, there can be no pain.

PAIN CHEMICALS

As soon as an injury occurs, the damaged cells begin to release three main pain chemicals. *Bradykinin*, the strongest pain-producing substance known, is responsible for starting the pain-message transmission. It is released when tiny blood vessels break in the damaged area. Nerve endings with special receptors for bradykinin begin sending pain messages as soon as the chemical is attached to them.

A second potent pain chemical is *substance P*, a protein that is released both at the injury site and in the spinal cord. Bradykinin starts pain; substance P keeps it going by reirritating the pain-sensing nerve endings at the spot where damage occurred. Substance P performs a similar job in the spinal cord: It keeps nerve tissues alert for pain messages.

A third chemical produced in reaction to bradykinin is prostaglandin, a hormone that draws infection-fighting cells to the site of injury or infection to help defend the body against disease-causing germs that could enter through a cut or burn. Prostaglandin also supplies fast help to the injury by making the body better able to send more pain messages and by causing them to flow faster. However, this has an unfortunate side effect: It makes the damaged area's nerve endings—and the injured individual—more sensitive to pain.

SIDE EFFECTS

The injury-site pain chemicals—bradykinin, substance P, and prostaglandin—are also responsible for the redness, warmth, and swelling of an injury. Bradykinin, for example, is a *vasodilator*, a substance that widens blood vessels in order to increase the blood supply. However, this also causes the injured area to redden, grow warmer, and swell. When bringing germ-fighting white cells to the area, prostaglandin also brings extra fluid. This increases the swelling, and the pressure of the swelling increases the pain.

Another substance, *histamine*, is sometimes released at an injury site. Histamine makes blood vessel walls more permeable, allowing fluid to leak out of them and cause further swelling in the surrounding area. The fluid carries infection-fighting cells. The purpose of this process is to defend the body against infectious germs.

STOP-PAIN SIGNALS

The brain reacts to pain messages by transmitting stop-pain signals back to the injury site. These signals travel down the spinal cord and

Along the pathway between the injury site and the brain, a pain message passes through a system of special pain receptor cells.

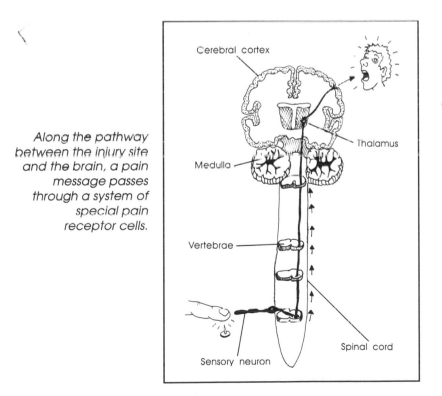

Cerebral cortex

Thalamus

Medulla

Vertebrae

Spinal cord

Sensory neuron

through the peripheral nervous system to the nerve cell that first received a nociceptor's pain signal. Grouped around the synapse between this first nerve cell and the second one are smaller nerve cells called *interneurons*. They function as gatekeepers to regulate the flow of pain messages from the site of the injury.

When stop-pain messages reach the end of an axon, they do not trigger the release of acetylcholine. Instead, neurotransmitters designed to stop pain, such as *norepinephrine* and *serotonin*, flow across the synapses and produce a different effect on the interneuron gatekeepers.

When norepinephrine is released into the synapse between the first and second nerve cells in the pain message route, it causes nearby interneurons to release molecules called *endorphins*, natural pain-relieving substances (similar to the painkilling drug *morphine*). The endorphins block the release of substance P from the injury. Without substance P, pain signals cannot be sent as efficiently by the first nerve cell to the second, which, at least partially, blocks the pain message.

When serotonin is released into the same synapse, it causes nearby interneurons to release a chemical called *gamma-aminobutyric acid*

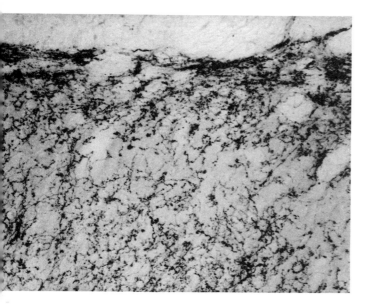

In this photograph of spinal cord tissue, the black, wavy structures are nerve endings that release serotonin, a neurotransmitter responsible for blocking pain signals before they reach the brain.

(GABA). GABA reduces the sensitivity of the second nerve cell in the chain, so it does not receive pain signals as efficiently. Again, the pain route is at least partially blocked.

INSIDE THE BRAIN

The brain's painkilling abilities depend on a different set of neuro-transmitters, called *enkephalins*. These chemicals are like the endorphins in their similarity to morphine, which is made from the opium poppy. In fact, their striking similarity to morphine is what led to the discovery of enkephalins.

Seeking to learn why morphine is such a powerful painkilling drug, scientists found special morphine receptors in parts of the brain that are important in relaying stop-pain signals to the body. But why, they wondered, would the brain have morphine receptors, when morphine is not a substance made by the body itself? How could such receptors have evolved? They concluded that the body must make its own morphinelike substances that attach to those receptors, and they soon found them. These chemicals turned out to be the endorphins and the enkephalins.

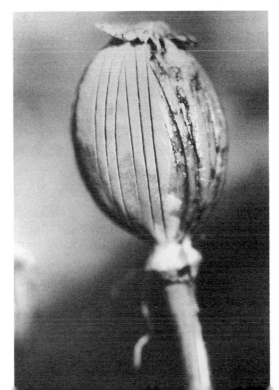

The brain manufactures its own natural painkilling substances that are similar to those found in morphine, a derivative of the poppy plant.

Within the brain, the *periaqueductal gray area* contains nerve cells studded with enkephalin receptors. Areas near these nerve cells contain a rich supply of the enkephalins themselves. Another section of the brain rich in receptors and enkephalins is the *locus coeruleus*, a nucleus in the brain stem. When either area receives pain signals from the reticular formation, it responds by releasing enkephalins into the receptors of its nerve cells. The enkephalins stimulate the cells to send the stop-pain chemicals, serotonin and norepinephrine, to the injury site. Once there, they stimulate GABA and the endorphins to block more pain messages from entering the nervous system.

Because of the body's complex and efficient pain-producing and pain-easing structures and chemicals, a minor injury may produce a pain that feels sudden and sharp yet diminishes quickly. However, this system does not work against every type of pain. Some injuries may be so severe and produce so many damage reports that the body's stop-pain system becomes overloaded. In other cases, a part of the nervous system itself is damaged by illness or injury and may keep sending pain signals even when no damage reports are coming in, or it may refuse to send or respond to stop-pain messages.

The brain short-circuits the whole stop-pain system when a lack of the brain's own pain-control enkephalins occurs. This shortage can happen when people who are addicted to morphine, *heroin*, or some other *opiate* suddenly stop taking the drugs. It occurs because the drugs fill up the brain's natural enkephalin receptors, so that normal enkephalins are no longer produced. When the drugs suddenly vanish from the brain, no enkephalins are ready to replace them; until the brain produces more natural enkephalins, the person has no stop-pain system at all. This is why it is painful, and sometimes actually dangerous, for an addict to abruptly stop taking drugs such as heroin or morphine. Physicians can provide a wide range of medicines to ease the pain of withdrawal and to make the process safe.

PAIN AND THE AUTONOMIC NERVOUS SYSTEM

Besides regulating pain itself, neurotransmitters also control many of the body's reactions to pain—the quickened heartbeat, faster breathing,

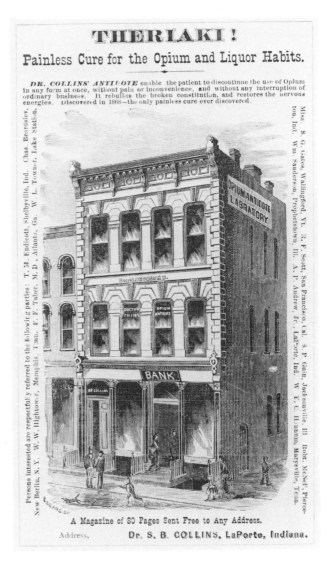

Addiction to opiates is not a new problem, but researchers are now able to explain its cause. When addicts use the drug often, it replaces the brain's natural production of pain relievers. When they quit using the drug, addicts suffer from withdrawal until their brains return to making the chemical naturally.

jitteriness, increased alertness, and other effects. Basically, the body has two nervous systems. The *voluntary nervous system* controls actions people consciously perform, such as walking and talking. The *autonomic nervous system* controls things the body does without thought, such as breathing, digesting food, and pumping blood.

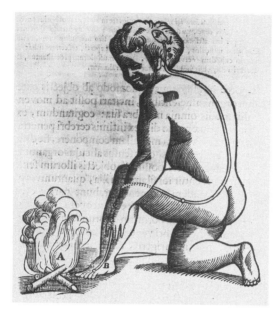

This 1677 illustration depicts science's early awareness of the body's autonomic nervous system, which is responsible for built-in responses to pain and other sensations.

When pain occurs, the brain sends messages through the nerves to prepare the whole body to act fast and forcefully to stop the pain's cause or to get away from it. The response makes the heart and breathing rates increase and the muscles tense. Hairs may stand up on the arms and the back of the neck, and the pupils of the eyes may dilate (widen) to let in more light. In addition, the senses may become extremely acute to hear or otherwise sense the cause of pain.

The cause of much of this intense readiness is *adrenaline*, a chemical released from the *adrenal glands*. These are a pair of wedge-shaped organs, each of which sits atop one of the kidneys. The brain signals the adrenal glands to release adrenaline in response to pain, strong emotion, or the perception of danger. The adrenaline traveling in the bloodstream raises heart and breathing rates, and as the heart pumps faster, blood pressure increases. This, in turn, raises blood sugar levels to provide sudden energy and to stimulate the senses. The adrenal glands also release substances called *corticosteroids*, hormones that make the body break down proteins to create even more energy and help maintain the body's water and chemical balance during times of pain or danger.

Once the danger or pain has passed, the autonomic nervous system uses acetylcholine, which is also active in the transmission of pain messages, to tell the body's automatic functions to relax. This dual purpose of acetylcholine demonstrates that the same chemical can serve very different purposes in different parts of the nervous system.

REFLEXES

In addition to helping the body get ready to combat or flee the cause of pain, the autonomic nervous system also helps the injured area avoid

Reflexes are part of the body's extremely fast response system to danger. When nerve cells in the spinal cord receive a pain message, they instantly send a message to the motor nerves, causing the muscles to react even before the brain becomes aware of the pain.

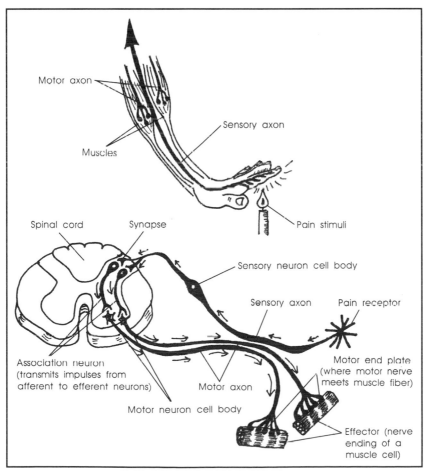

43

pain as quickly as possible. For instance, when a person touches a hot stove, he or she jerks back instantaneously—before the sensation of pain can register in the brain. Although the pain arrives in a short time, how can the body react before the pain message is received by the brain?

The answer is in the *reflexes*, the body's extremely fast reaction system. When a pain message is received by certain nerve cells in the spinal cord, they transmit the message back to *motor nerves* (nerves that control muscle movement) near the injury site. Before even the brain receives the message, the motor nerves send to the muscles signals that provoke an instantaneous response to avoid the source of pain. Any action performed automatically in response to a stimulus is called a *reflex action*.

Pain messages are not the only ones to cause reflex actions. An object moving rapidly toward the eye will cause it to blink by reflex, or a tap on just the right spot on the knee will cause the leg to jerk up, also by reflex. Because reflexes occur before the brain even receives the messages that provoke the response, a person cannot choose whether or not to have a reflexive response.

The body's ability to sense and react to pain depends on a complex system of structures and substances. The types of pain are equally varied and complex in response to the many kinds of injuries and illnesses that can cause them. The next chapter examines the varieties of pain and investigates some unsolved pain mysteries that continue to puzzle scientists.

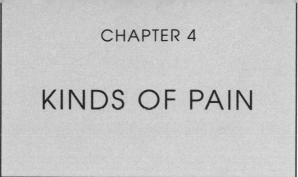

CHAPTER 4

KINDS OF PAIN

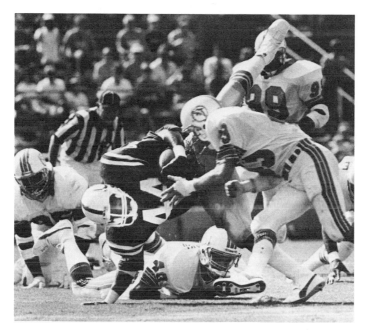

Pain is experienced in many ways. The players in this 1986 game between the Indianapolis Colts and the Miami Dolphins were probably so involved in the action that they did not feel much pain until the game was over.

Most people can recall having an injury that seems severe, perhaps a bloody cut or a broken bone. Such wounds are so unusual and unexpected that they create a feeling of shock and fear—which only makes the injury hurt even more. Yet a short visit to the doctor or infirmary may soon soothe these worries, and suddenly the pain is barely noticeable.

The varieties of misery people feel are as numerous as the causes of pain. And as mentioned earlier, pain is often influenced by thoughts and feelings. Pain caused by a broken leg may be severe, but it goes away as the injury heals; knowing it will go away helps it seem less severe. By contrast, long-lasting pain may feel less intense, yet cause more suffering because the constant, nagging pain wears down the ability to bear the discomfort. Fear makes a pain hurt more, while knowing an injury is not dangerous can make it hurt less.

A person's cultural background can also affect the pain he or she experiences. An individual who learns from family and friends that the normal response to pain is great suffering and distress tends to feel that distress, whereas a person from an environment where pain is ignored tends to experience less discomfort. Good news, the presence of friends, a gloomy day, or a shortage of money can all change the way people experience pain. The statement, My pain is different from anyone else's, is the truth: Each person's pain is uniquely his or her own.

ACUTE PAIN

Individual pains can be grouped into categories, according to shared traits. One major type of pain is *acute pain*, which is sudden, sharp, and short-lived. The cause may be as simple as a stubbed toe, or as

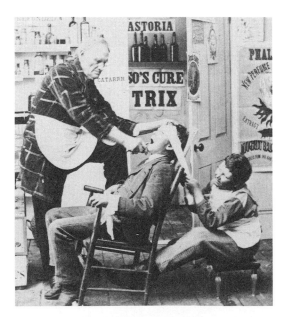

Acute pain, such as a toothache, appears suddenly and usually ends quickly. Often it signals a problem that needs immediate care and disappears as soon as it is treated.

serious as a broken leg, bad burn, or head injury. In any case, acute pain makes the body want to combat or escape the cause. The whole body joins in this effort by means of the secondary effects of acute pain: fast heartbeat, fast breathing, heightened senses, and all of the body's *fight-or-flight* preparations. (These preparations are the body's automatic response to stress or anxiety, enabling an individual to flee or defend him- or herself from potential danger.)

Acute pain disappears quickly in response to the body's system for sending pain and stop-pain messages. Autonomic reflexes intercept the pain messages and react instantly by sending the stop-pain chemicals to block pain messages almost at their source. This prevents them from traveling any farther through the nervous system toward the brain.

CHRONIC PAIN

Chronic pain is different from acute pain because it does not go away for a long time. For this reason, it may be a warning signal of an unhealed injury or disease. For example, arthritis, an ailment of the joints that produces swelling and tenderness, may cause pain that comes back day after day, for weeks, months, or years. On the other hand, chronic pain may be a false alarm. For example, pain nerves can become stuck, acting like a broken switch that cannot be turned off. Long after an illness is over or an injury is healed, those nerves keep sending pain messages to the brain even though there is no ongoing damage to produce them.

In their book *Pain Control*, pain specialists Bruce Smoller, M.D. of the George Washington School of Medicine and Brian Schulman, M.D. of the Georgetown University School of Medicine say that millions of Americans suffer chronic pain so severe that many are unable to work, go to school, or socialize. The doctors estimate that 5 million are disabled by back pain, with a total of 40 million Americans who suffer from chronic headaches and other chronic pains.

Unlike acute pain sufferers, who know that the pain will go away when their illness or injury heals, chronic-pain victims endure not only today's misery but the knowledge that tomorrow, next week, and even next year could be as painful as the present moment. As a result, a

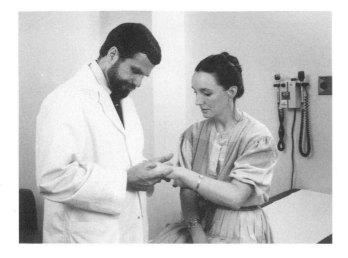

Individuals who suffer from chronic pain often visit one doctor after another, finding that none of them can offer long-term solutions to the problem.

chronic sufferer may go from one doctor to the next, searching for one who can relieve the pain, and undergoing numerous tests and repeated surgeries in the vain hope that something will help. He or she may become addicted to painkilling drugs, which work less effectively as the body grows accustomed to them. The patient's friends and family may tire of hearing about the chronic pain, and his or her doctors may even lose sympathy, especially if no physical cause can be pinpointed.

Eventually, some people may suggest that the individual is faking pain to avoid work or school or to get sympathy or special treatment. Others may believe the discomfort is all in the patient's head or become angry and frustrated at their own inability to help. To avoid such attitudes, the chronic-pain victim may spend more time alone.

Finally, chronic pain becomes a vicious circle, as negative thoughts and feelings make the pain worse, and the increased pain in turn makes the thoughts and feelings more unhappy. Soon the person's entire existence can deteriorate, a condition known as *chronic pain syndrome*.

This problem has no quick cure because often the pain cannot be completely eliminated. Yet doctors who specialize in caring for people suffering from this syndrome can combine painkilling drugs and other therapies with a program of attitude-and-behavior modification to get the person off the "chronic pain merry-go-round." Such a program often involves family members because they, too, are affected by the

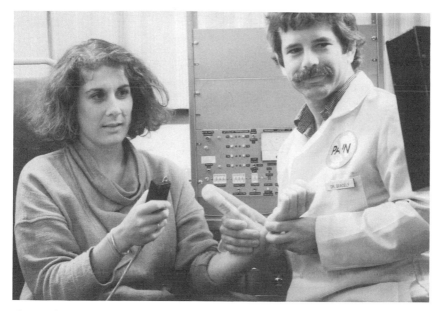

A psychologist at the National Institutes of Health (NIH) Pain Research Clinic in Bethesda, Maryland, applies thermal stimulation to a patient's arm while the patient uses a monitor to select words describing the sensations she feels. Understanding a person's reactions to pain is an important part of pain research.

pain, and their feelings and behavior toward it can help make the situation better or worse. With such treatment a chronic pain victim can stop being a victim and return to a satisfying life even when some pain still exists.

Neuralgia

A specific kind of chronic pain is *neuralgia*, pain caused by damage to nerves in the peripheral nervous system. Neuralgia causes a nerve damaged by infection or injury to send pain messages in response to things that are not ordinarily painful, such as a light touch or the normal activity of chewing food. Sometimes, a nerve may begin sending pain messages all by itself. Neuralgic pain is intense and may spread; for instance, touching the hand might make the whole arm hurt. Scientists do not know exactly how or why neuralgic pain occurs, but they do know that viruses—such as *herpes zoster* ("shingles"), which is related to the virus that causes chicken pox—vitamin deficiencies, poor circulation, and some poisons, such as arsenic, can cause neuralgias. In some cases, though, the cause is unidentified.

Injections of anesthetic drugs sometimes soothe neuralgic pain for a while. They are injected either into the nerves linked to the injured area or into ganglia near the spinal cord. One promising method of relief encourages the nerves to switch pain signals for a different message by stimulating them with a tiny electrical current. Called *transcutaneous electrical nerve stimulation* (TENS), the technique relieves certain types of neuralgia and some other kinds of chronic pain in about half of all patients treated. Even when the technique does work, however, the nerves seem to adjust to the current over a period of months and begin once again to send pain messages.

Causalgia

Causalgia is another type of chronic pain that arises from damage to nerves. It occurs in 2% to 5% of those people who suffer bullet or stab wounds to peripheral nerves. Very severe and burning, the pain persists even after the wound has healed. In 85% of cases it lasts longer than 6 months, and in 25% it lasts a year or more. Causalgia involves not only the pain nerves but also the autonomic nerves, those that control automatic body functions, such as sweating and blood circulation, in the affected area.

A gentle touch, a bright light, or even a sudden thought or emotion can bring on the torture of causalgia. Yet keeping the affected area still only makes things worse: Reducing normal movement and sensation seems to train the brain to keep feeling pain, so that eventually even amputating the affected part does not stop the misery. Some patients with causalgia can retrain the nerves and brain to stop transmitting pain signals by gradually increasing sensations to the problem area. For example, a patient may first put the affected part in water, then in running water, then have it massaged, and so on. Other causalgia sufferers need injections of nerve-numbing drugs into the spinal cord, or a type of nerve surgery called a *sympathectomy* to cut or remove the autonomic nerves in the area.

PHANTOM PAIN

Phantom pain occurs in a body part that no longer exists, such as an amputated arm, hand, leg, or foot. Although the limb is no longer attached to the body, it feels as though it is still there—and continues to hurt. Most people who have undergone amputation agree that in the beginning they receive sensations that feel as if the part is still there. They may reach out for something with an absent arm or try to walk on a foot no longer present.

The sensation of phantom pain is similar to the one that occurs after the dentist administers a shot of local anesthetic: The numbed lip feels fat and swollen, even though it is not swollen at all. The numbed lip is not sending any nerve signals to the brain, and in response to the lack of signals, the brain apparently fabricates sensations that should be there.

In most people the brain gradually accepts that the amputated limb is gone, and the phantom sensation fades. But it persists either con-

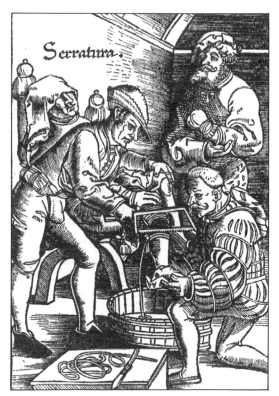

Amputations have been performed for centuries, as shown in this 1517 picture in the Field-Book of Wound Surgery. However, amputation does not always ensure that the pain will cease. Phantom pain refers to discomfort sensed in missing limbs.

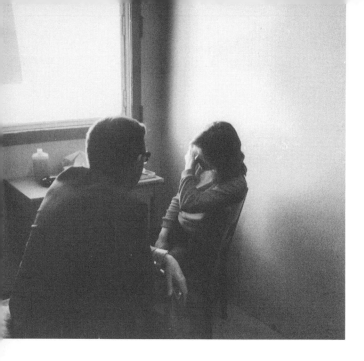

People who suffer from psychogenic pain consider it real, although medical tests can find no cause for the problem. Treatment often involves the expertise of psychologists.

stantly or intermittently in about 5% of amputees, though scientists do not fully understand why. Injections of nerve-numbing drugs often relieve the pain, yet it tends to recur and the injections must be repeated.

PSYCHOGENIC PAIN

Psychogenic pain is similar to chronic pain: It is long-lasting and tends to undermine the quality of life. Psychogenic pain may be felt in the head, back, or elsewhere but is not caused by a physical ailment. Instead, the source can be severe depression or other emotional or mental disorders.

Psychogenic pain is not a fake sensation: People who suffer from it are experiencing real pain. Even so, drugs, surgery, or other pain relief techniques do not help. Only treating the mental and emotional causes of the pain (through therapy for example) will ease the problem.

Most people will never suffer from chronic, phantom, or psychogenic pain. Yet everyone has encountered acute pain that, though sudden, usually ends quickly. The next chapter discusses some of the more common pains, examining why such pains occur, what can be done about them, which ones tend not to be serious, and which ones should be brought to the attention of a physician at once.

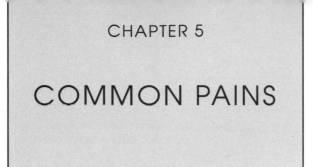

CHAPTER 5

COMMON PAINS

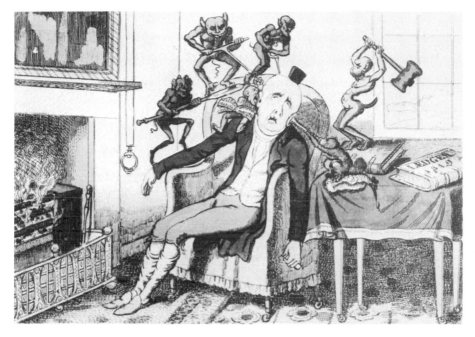

Headaches are probably the most common pain people experience. Yet not every headache feels the same, because their causes vary widely.

Pain is the most common medical symptom people experience, according to the National Institutes of Health. It indicates that an individual may have a physical disorder requiring medical attention. So the ability to evaluate pain—to decide whether or not its cause is serious and what to do about it—is extremely important.

The severity of a pain—how much it hurts—can be a good clue to its seriousness. A truly agonizing pain, especially one that has not occurred in the past, that comes on all at once, and that does not go away or keeps returning, is a strong warning signal. Yet severity alone is not always a cause for worry. For instance, a minor burn hurts a lot but usually is not dangerous. As important as the amount of pain that occurs is the quality of the pain: Is it sharp, dull, grinding, heavy, or shooting? A tension headache that feels like a band tightened around the head can make a person miserable but normally is not a signal of anything seriously wrong. By contrast, a sudden thunderclap head pain can mean a blood vessel has burst in the brain. When it hurts is also important: A headache experienced while a person has a cold or the flu is probably just a flu symptom, but a headache experienced in the hours or days after a blow to the head may signal serious injury.

Where a pain hurts can also be important. A pain in the right lower abdomen, for instance, often signals appendicitis and the need for immediate surgery. In contrast, a pain in the lower back is more likely to mean muscle strain and the need for rest and aspirin. Symptoms experienced along with pain are important too: A stiff neck by itself can mean a minor muscle cramp, but with a high fever it may signal a brain infection.

HEADACHES

Headache is one of the most common pains suffered by young adults. In fact, according to the National Center for Health Statistics, this complaint causes children and teens to miss a total of 1.3 million school days per year. The causes of headache range from simple and non-dangerous—the anxiety of an upcoming exam or sports tryout, for instance, or eye fatigue after a long study session—to complex and even life-threatening.

A common type of headache, called a *tension* or *muscle-contraction headache*, feels like a dull, heavy, or pressing pain on both sides of the head and in the neck, yet it normally signals no danger. Some people seldom experience them and find help in rest and perhaps a mild pain reliever such as aspirin. Others have severe tension headaches that can last continuously for days or months.

Scientists do not yet know the precise physical cause for tension headaches, but a 1980 study reported in the medical journal *Pain*

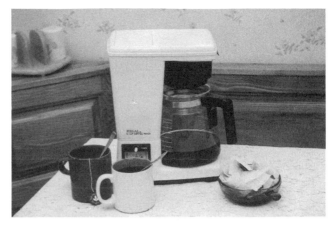

Vascular headaches may be induced by consuming drinks containing caffeine, such as coffee, tea, and cola, or foods with too many chemical preservatives. Such substances cause blood vessels in the brain to widen, creating a pounding pain.

suggests that some people who have frequent or chronic episodes may be unusually sensitive to histamine, one of the body's important pain chemicals. In addition, a 1981 study reported in the medical journal *Headache* suggests that sufferers of frequent tension headaches may be deficient in one of the brain's pain-regulating substances, serotonin. If tension headaches occur often, the sufferer should visit a physician to determine the cause, to learn how to prevent them if possible, and to get help for the pain.

Vascular Headaches

Some people get *vascular headaches*, which are characterized by pounding or thudding pain. They arise when blood vessels in the brain become dilated (widened) and send pain messages as a result of the abnormal stretching of their walls. Such headaches can be caused by foods containing *nitrites* (chemical preservatives), such as hot dogs, salami, and bacon, and by the chemical *monosodium glutamate* (MSG), a flavor-enhancing additive. Drinking too much of caffeine-laden beverages, such as coffee, tea, or cola, can cause vascular headaches in some people, and imbibing too much alcohol will have the same effect on almost anyone. Vascular headaches caused by food-additive sensitivities are often prevented by avoiding the offending foods.

For some people, exercise causes vascular headaches. This occurs when the heart rate increases, sending extra blood through the vessels. In response, the vessels widen a tiny amount to accept the extra blood

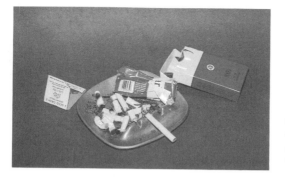

About 1 in 40 Americans, mostly male cigarette smokers, are afflicted by cluster headaches. This especially painful condition, usually accompanied by other uncomfortable symptoms, often appears first during the teen years.

flow; the stretch triggers the headache. Exercise-induced headaches can be prevented with prescribed medicines that are taken only before exercise sessions.

A severe type of vascular headache is the *cluster headache*, an agonizing pain occurring on just one side of the head and accompanied by a variety of symptoms, including sweating, tearing of the eyes, and blurred vision. Most sufferers are men, and almost all are cigarette smokers. People who get cluster headaches—about 1 in 40 Americans—have them repeatedly. Often, the first one occurs during the teen years. Breathing pure oxygen stops the pain in 80% of the cases; 75% of the remaining cases respond to drugs.

An isolated, pounding headache with a known cause—the sufferer's having drunk too much coffee, for instance, or having eaten certain foods—is not likely to signal a serious problem. However, a severe pounding headache that does not go away, or keeps recurring, accompanied by other symptoms, deserves the attention of a physician. A doctor may help rule out serious causes, prevent more headaches, and relieve the pain.

Migraine Headaches

Migraine headaches, which also recur on just one side of the head, are suffered by about 25 million people in the United States alone. These headaches consist of violent throbbing pain, often accompanied by nausea and extreme sensitivity to light. They may also cause the patient to perceive *auras*, sensations made of sounds, smells, and patterns of colored light, none of which are actually present. A survey in the Danish medical journal *Clinical Aspects of Migraine* reported that by age 19, 19% of young women and 11% of young men suffer migraines, and that about 60% of them will continue having the headaches through later life.

The causes of migraine are not well understood by doctors, and there is no certain cure, although some sufferers are helped by drugs and other treatments. Although a migraine headache is not dangerous in itself, migraine sufferers should be examined by a physician to ensure that the headache is really a migraine, rather than a warning sign of a more serious condition.

A few headache symptoms are real danger signals. The following list describes symptoms indicating an immediate need for medical attention:

- A sudden, extremely painful headache that appears out of nowhere and feels like a thunderclap inside the head. This may signal a burst or leaking blood vessel in the brain, which can be life threatening.

- A headache accompanied by numbness, weakness, twitching, or *convulsions* (fits or seizures). These symptoms may signal an infection or injury in the brain or nervous system

- A headache with fever, when a person is not ill with a cold or the flu. This may indicate an infection in the brain or spinal cord.

- A headache accompanied by confusion, loss of consciousness, or odd behavior. This may signal a number of serious conditions deserving immediate medical attention.

- A headache accompanied by a pain in the eye or ear, or a stiff neck. This discomfort may indicate an infection or other disorder.

- Recurrent headaches in children, or a sudden change in a child's headache. These may signal a serious illness. Children's headaches come from serious causes more often than those of teens or adults.

An individual who suddenly develops recurring headaches should be examined. The problem may not necessitate a race to the emergency room, but the cause should eventually be determined by a doctor. By the same token, headaches that occur when an individual coughs, stoops, or strains; that awaken a person at night; or that interfere with a person's daily activities are not always danger signs but should be investigated.

Headaches that occur after a blow to the head, whether they occur immediately or days to weeks after the injury, must be evaluated by a physician. These headaches are not always serious, but some may signal brain damage that only a physician can diagnose.

Drinking too much alcohol often results in a vascular headache. This 1883 wood engraving illustrates a variety of dangers brought on by absinthe, a popular liquor at that time.

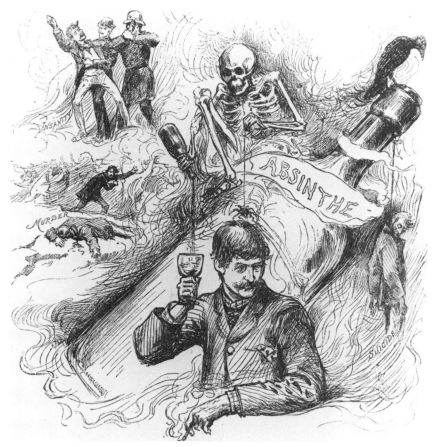

OTHER HEAD PAINS

Three nonheadache pains that occur in the area of the head are eye pain, toothache, and ear pain. These pains usually signal the need for treatment. Any sudden severe pain in the eye should be checked by a physician at once, since it may indicate infection or some other vision-destroying ailment. A toothache is often a sign of a cavity or an infected tooth; prompt treatment will not only stop the pain but also keep any possible infection from spreading into the jaw or the rest of the body. Ear pain often signals an ear infection, which requires treatment with antibiotics to stop pain and prevent hearing loss. Like headaches, sore throats can result from a wide variety of causes and are rarely a sign of a serious problem. Often they are a symptom of a minor illness, such as a cold, the flu, or a virus that will clear up by itself in a day or so. However, a few sore throats are symptoms of ailments requiring a doctor's help. A sore throat that is red with white spots is a sign of infection by the *streptococcus* bacteria. Often called *strep throat*, this condition, once diagnosed, should be treated with antibiotics to stop the pain and prevent the infection from spreading.

A very sore, red throat with no white spots, sometimes accompanied by headache, swollen glands, fatigue, or an overall poor feeling may signal *mononucleosis*, a viral infection most prevalent among young adults. Known colloquially as *mono*, the condition usually needs no drug treatment, but the patient should see a doctor because the ailment can have serious complications in some cases.

A sore throat that has a white or yellow coating can signal *tonsillitis* (a bacterial infection of the tonsils), especially if the person also has a fever. Infected tonsils should be treated by a doctor, who will probably prescribe antibiotics against the infection. Any sore throat that does not go away within 48 hours, is accompanied by a high fever, or is painful enough to prevent swallowing should be seen by a doctor to determine the cause and treatment.

STOMACH PAIN

Stomach pains can come from a variety of causes ranging from the minor (too much ice cream or a touch of stomach flu) to the extremely

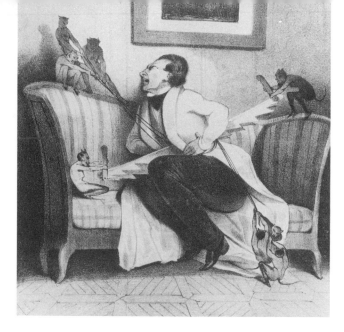

serious (an infected or burst appendix or a ruptured spleen). It is not possible to detail all of the causes of stomach pain, but it can be useful to follow a few guidelines when evaluating them.

If a person experiences pain in the upper left part of the abdomen after falling hard, being in an auto accident, or suffering a solid body blow (while playing sports, for example), he or she may have suffered a ruptured spleen. This injury needs immediate medical attention.

If an individual has pain in the lower right portion of the abdomen or directly around the navel (belly button) that lasts for more than 12 hours, he or she may have appendicitis. A doctor should be consulted at once.

A sudden, severe, unfamiliar pain in any part of the stomach or abdomen that lasts for 30 minutes or more is another danger signal requiring immediate attention.

If a female thinks there is any chance that she may be pregnant and she experiences sudden severe pain in the lower abdomen, she should see a physician immediately. She may have a condition called *ruptured ectopic pregnancy*, which is brought on by the disruption of an abnormal type of pregnancy that occurs outside the uterus and requires immediate surgery.

Women also suffer frequently from *menstrual pain*, aching or cramps in the abdomen during menstruation that, though uncomfortable, are not dangerous. For reasons that doctors do not completely understand, some women have little or no pain during this time while others have discomfort severe enough to prevent them from going to work or school. Menstrual pain intense enough to interfere with a woman's daily life should be brought to a doctor's attention not only to make sure it has no other cause but because simple and effective pain relief is available for most severe menstrual pain. Often the drug ibuprofen is used.

Another medical problem that is directly related to menstruation is *premenstrual syndrome*, or PMS, which occurs for various amounts of time prior to menstrual bleeding. Its symptoms range from fatigue and depression to constipation, backaches, and pimples. Most women experience this discomfort at some time or another, while about 40% encounter it regularly. Treatment includes special diets, vitamins, exercises, and, in severe cases, hormone treatments.

If a person knows why he or she is having stomach pain, then the pain probably does not need treatment. This includes when a person eats or drinks too much, eats something that does not agree with him or her, or gets a stomach ache when nervous but not at any other time. If a pain is mild, goes away by itself, and does not come back, then it usually is no cause for concern.

However, if the pain is severe, does not go away, or goes away but keeps coming back, then a physician should be consulted to find the pain's cause and relieve the discomfort.

BODY PAIN

Back pains, muscle pains, and joint pains come from a variety of causes ranging from the minor to the serious.

Perhaps the most common cause of minor aches and pains is exercise. Everyone knows how it feels to wake up stiff and sore the day after the first big game of the season or after a long hike or bicycle ride: The joints and muscles have suddenly done a lot of work they are not used to, and they protest—painfully. Easing the common pains that occur after vigorous exercise is usually just a matter of a hot shower, gentle movement to loosen the muscles, and perhaps an aspirin or two.

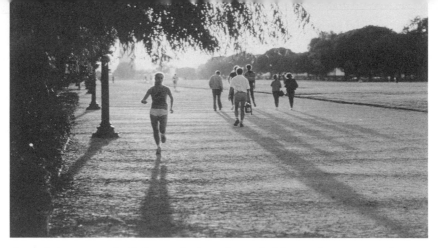

A certain amount of discomfort, such as slight muscle soreness, is normal during or after exercise. But precautions, such as stretching gently and moving properly, should be taken to avoid sudden and severe strain.

Some exercise-related pains are avoidable, however, if the proper clothing and equipment are used. For example, it is wise to wear a shoe with good support and plenty of cushioning for walking or running. Beating pain also requires taking the appropriate steps to get in shape. A program of conditioning might involve, a few weeks of short daily bicycle rides before setting out on a 15-mile bike trip. Each time a person exercises, he or she should prepare gradually for more strenuous exercise. For instance, a runner can avoid sprains and pulls by gently stretching the leg muscles before running.

Learning the proper form for the kind of exercise or physical work undertaken also prevents aches and pains. For example, bending from the waist to lift a heavy box is almost certain to strain the muscles of the back, resulting in pain and possibly permanent injury. But if a person bends at the knees and lifts with a straight back, the leg muscles will do most of the lifting, which preserves the back muscles.

Back, joint, or muscle pain that occurs after more exercise than a person is accustomed to but that is not severe and goes away in a few days is not usually a signal of anything seriously wrong. If such pains are very severe (especially those intense enough to keep a person from work or school) or are accompanied by redness, swelling, fever, or similar symptoms, medical help should be sought.

In addition, back, muscle, or joint pains that occur during exercise or result from any kind of injury should be seen by a physician if they hurt a great deal and do not go away in a short time. Such pains may be a sign of a torn muscle or a damaged *ligament* or *cartilage*, connective tissues that hold the bones in line. They may even signal an undetected broken bone.

Back or neck pain accompanied by numbness or tingling in an injured body part should be seen by a doctor at once, as it may signal nerve or spinal cord damage. If such symptoms occur immediately after an accident or sports injury, the victim should not be moved except by trained emergency medical technicians. Otherwise, damage to the spinal cord may cause permanent paralysis.

CHEST PAIN

Like other pains, chest pain can signal ailments and injuries ranging from trivial muscle strains to life-threatening medical emergencies such as heart attacks or punctured lungs. Generally, anyone can experience a heart attack, so everyone should know the signs of a heart attack and what to do if one occurs. In an adult, any sudden chest pain with an unknown cause should be treated as a possible heart attack. The person should be seen by a doctor at once, especially if the pain feels heavy or pressing, radiates to the left arm, shoulder, or jaw, and includes faintness, shortness of breath, or palpitations. In young adults, the chance of a chest pain signaling a heart attack is slim, but it can happen, especially in those who abuse drugs. One cause of chest pains that young adults get, although rarely, is *spontaneous pneumothorax*, a hole in one of the tiny air sacs in the lungs. When this occurs, air leaks from the lung into the space between the lung and the chest wall. The main symptom is sudden, unexplained shortness of breath, sometimes accompanied by sharp chest pain that does not go away. Although doctors do not know why some otherwise perfectly healthy young people—most of them men—suffer spontaneous pneumothorax, they do know how to repair the damage: Surgery is needed immediately to patch the leak.

Chest pain occurring with each breath can be due to infections of the lungs or the lining of the chest wall. If the pain occurs only when a person coughs, and he or she has a cold or the flu, the pain could be caused simply by sore muscles from frequent coughing. However, a doctor should be consulted if the pain is severe enough to interfere with breathing, if it is accompanied by a high fever, or if the cough produces either blood or green, yellow, or brown sputum (mucus). In addition, any chest pain whose cause is not obvious, such as muscle soreness or a minor bruise, and that does not go away in a few days should be brought to a doctor's attention. Of course, after a blow or injury to the chest, any severe or lasting chest pain should be seen by a doctor, since it may signal a cracked or broken rib.

INTERNAL PAIN

A pain that many young adults find embarrassing to talk about, but one that is common and usually easy to cure, is pain during urination. This is sometimes accompanied by blood in the urine, and the cause is almost always a bacterial infection of the *bladder*, the organ that collects urine, or of the *urethra*, the tube that carries urine out of the body. Antibiotics prescribed by a physician can get rid of the infection and pain very quickly. However, if a person does not receive treatment, the infection can spread to and damage the kidneys, so the problem should always be brought to the attention of a doctor right away. Moreover, in some cases, urination accompanied by pain and blood can be a sign of a damaged kidney or bladder, requiring immediate treatment. This particularly applies to a person who has suffered a blow to the abdomen or to the *flank*, the middle part of the back, toward the side. Similarly, any other pain, sores, or discharge in the genital area should receive prompt medical care.

Many pains exist other than those mentioned in this chapter. Fortunately, most are not severe, dangerous, or a sign of a serious problem. For pain that does need medical treatment, young people and others may take comfort in the fact that medical help is available from school nurses, family doctors, medical clinics, and the staff of hospital emergency rooms—all dedicated to treating illnesses, healing injuries, and relieving the many varieties of pain. If a person feels doubt about the nature of an ongoing pain, he or she should not hesitate to seek help.

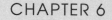

CHAPTER 6

DRUGS TO TREAT PAIN

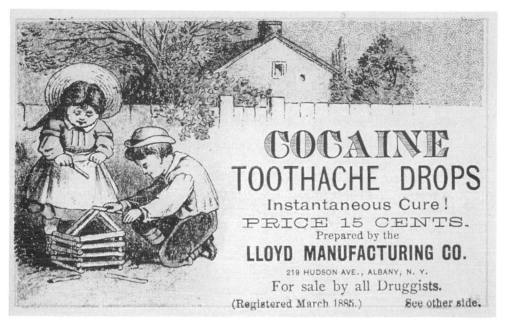

COCAINE
TOOTHACHE DROPS
Instantaneous Cure!
PRICE 15 CENTS.
Prepared by the
LLOYD MANUFACTURING CO.
219 HUDSON AVE., ALBANY, N. Y.
For sale by all Druggists.
(Registered March 1885.)   See other side.

Drug manufacturers often promise an instantaneous cure. Although there are no magic cure-alls, people should learn which medicines are available and the appropriate times to use them.

Twentieth-century science and medicine have provided more numerous and effective drugs for pain relief than ever before. The latest edition of the *Physician's Desk Reference* lists more than 165 separate substances that form the active ingredients in thousands of pain-relieving medications available by prescription. According to the U.S. Food and Drug Administration (FDA), among the over-the-counter (nonprescription) drugs for pain relief, more than 50,000

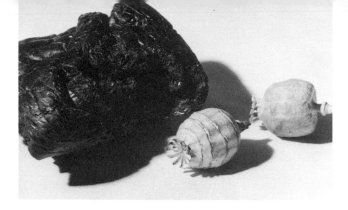

Derived from opium, an extract of the poppy plant, narcotics have provided a primary source of pain relief for several millennia. They still seem to offer the greatest relief for severe pain.

products are based on the active ingredient in aspirin. Thousands more are based on similar drugs, such as acetaminophen and ibuprofen.

The number and variety of over-the-counter pain remedies available, and the amount of advertising they receive, can be confusing. Some people think they can find a pill for every pain, either from the drugstore or the doctor. Fast relief from a drug has become the first and often the only thing these people think of when they have pain. Others, due to current concerns about the dangers of illicit drugs, avoid all pain-relieving drugs even when it might be appropriate to take them. An unrealistic fear of getting hooked causes some people to suffer needless pain.

By contrast, good pain relief choices are based on clear thinking and knowledge about drugs and how they work, their effectiveness on different kinds of pain, and especially their side effects, the unwanted effects all drugs have in addition to the desired ones.

Drugs that travel through the bloodstream must also be metabolized—broken down by the liver into simpler substances, then sent by carrier proteins formed in the liver to the area where they are effective. After a drug has performed its job, the excess, along with the waste products formed when the drug is broken down by the liver, must be excreted—filtered out of the bloodstream by the kidneys and liver, and removed from the body in the form of urine (liquid waste) or feces (solid waste).

NARCOTICS

The two main categories of pain-relieving drugs are the *narcotics* and the *non-narcotics*. The narcotic drugs, derived from an extract of the opium poppy, have been used for thousands of years to relieve severe pain. Narcotics seem to be the most effective drugs against severe pain, including the discomfort brought on by serious illnesses or major surgery.

The naturally derived narcotics, also called opiates, include morphine, *codeine*, and the illegal drug heroin. More recently discovered, synthetic narcotics are made by altering natural narcotics in the laboratory to make them longer lasting or to decrease their side effects. Synthetic narcotics, called *opioids* to distinguish them from naturally derived drugs, include Dilaudid, methadone, *Demerol*, *Talwin*, and *Percodan*.

Whether natural or synthetic, narcotics are available only by prescription because they can be habit-forming. They relieve pain by acting on the central nervous system—the brain, the spinal cord, or both. Hence, their side effects include drowsiness, apathy, slowed breathing, lowered concentration, and general slowing of all the body functions controlled by the nervous system. Overdose of a narcotic can cause respiratory failure, coma, and death.

All narcotics relieve pain in the same general way. Their molecular structure is so much like that of the brain's own natural painkilling

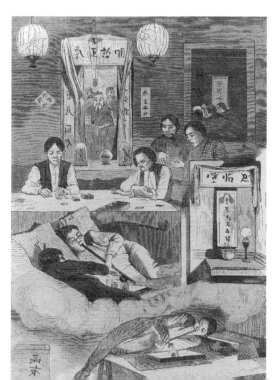

This 1874 wood engraving of a New York opium den illustrates the unfortunate side effect of narcotics—addiction. In recent decades, researchers have developed synthetic narcotics, which are less addictive and longer lasting.

molecules, called endorphins, that the narcotic molecules can attach themselves to endorphin-receptor sites in the brain. When the receptor sites are filled—with endorphins or the endorphinlike narcotics—the brain's ability to experience pain becomes dulled. The sensation itself is still there, but the brain simply fails to recognize the sensation as pain. The person experiencing the sensation no longer finds it unpleasant. This describes the condition of *analgesia*—the removal not of a sensation, but of its painful quality. Hence, narcotics are *analgesic drugs*.

The way narcotics work—by substituting for the brain's own pain-relief molecules—is also the reason that narcotics are so habit-forming. When the brain is regularly supplied with narcotic molecules, it stops making its own supply of natural endorphins. Then, when the supply of narcotics is cut off, the brain is left with no pain-relieving molecules at all—a condition that allows pain messages to flood the brain, causing misery to the addicted person until he or she takes more narcotic drugs. However, if no more narcotic drugs are taken, the brain eventually will begin producing more endorphins, easing the pain of drug withdrawal. Yet the craving for narcotics may persist even after withdrawal pains are gone.

Narcotic drugs have drawbacks beyond their addictive qualities. The brain tends to get used to them, so that after a while they do not relieve pain as well. In addition, their tendency to cause drowsiness prevents a person taking them from participating in activities such as driving a car, working, and studying. As a result, narcotic drugs are reserved for the very severe types of pain that require them. Against lesser or chronic pains, non-narcotic drugs are a safer and more useful choice.

NON-NARCOTIC ANALGESICS

The pain-relieving drugs used by most people to treat common pains, such as headaches, muscle pains, backache, and toothache, are the non-narcotic analgesics. Like narcotic analgesics, they block pain but do not produce numbness. Unlike the narcotics, however, they do not work in the central nervous system, and thus they do not have many of

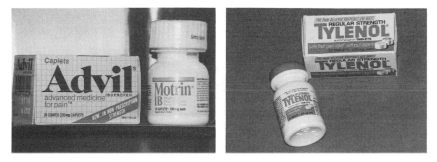

Non-narcotic analgesics offer the best help for common pains, easing discomfort at the site where it occurs. Although aspirin is the best-known analgesic, acetaminophen, sold under names such as Tylenol and Datril, and ibuprofen, marketed as Nuprin and Advil, work in similar ways and with fewer side effects.

the undesirable side effects of narcotic pain drugs, such as addictiveness. This permits non-narcotic analgesics to be sold over the counter. The main non-narcotic analgesics—aspirin, acetaminophen, and ibuprofen—work directly at the site where pain signals originate—for instance, at the throbbing tooth, inflamed joint, or sore muscle.

Aspirin, acetaminophen, and ibuprofen work against pain in similar ways. They stop injured tissues from producing prostaglandins, substances that make an injury become red and swollen and that sensitize the nerve endings so they receive and send messages more efficiently. Thus, aspirin, acetaminophen, and ibuprofen are effective against pains produced by the substance prostaglandin, such as headache, toothache, and muscle soreness. However, they are not useful when prostaglandin release is not involved in the pain. For instance, if a person took two aspirin and was then stuck by a pin, the aspirin would not block the sudden stab of pain, which would be transmitted to the brain long before the prostaglandins were released. Yet the aspirin will later ease the redness, soreness, and swelling of the injury.

Over-the-counter non-narcotic analgesics are safe and effective for most people when used as directed. Yet, like all drugs, they do have some side effects. This particularly applies to aspirin, which can irritate the stomach and so should be taken with milk or food. Aspirin also increases the time it takes for blood to clot, which means it could be harmful to people who are also taking blood-thinning medicines or to people with bleeding problems. Additionally, people who are allergic to aspirin should not take it under any circumstances. They should instead ask their doctors for advice on what pain remedy is safe for them to take.

In children and young adults, aspirin has been associated with an increase in severe complications from Reye's syndrome, an often fatal disease of the brain characterized by fever, vomiting, and swelling of the kidneys and brain. It is recommended that young people with flulike illnesses use nonaspirin remedies, rather than aspirin. Moreover, taking too many aspirin can cause stomach bleeding, kidney or liver damage, and even death.

ADJUVANT AGENTS

Barbiturates, *tranquilizers* (drugs known for their ability to create a calm mental state), and marijuana act much as narcotic analgesics do: They work directly on the central nervous system to relieve pain but do not stop the sensation altogether. These drugs are called *adjuvants* because they can be used to intensify the actions of stronger drugs while producing fewer side effects. They also help a patient undergoing surgery by easing the emotional stress and anxiety that tend to increase pain. In recent years, researchers have reported that marijuana also helps combat the nausea and loss of appetite that generally accompany chemotherapy and AIDS. Although the adjuvants are not narcotics, they can be addictive and require prescriptions.

ANESTHETICS

Anesthetics are also non-narcotic drugs. They differ from the analgesics because they do not merely remove the painfulness of a sensation but block the entire sensation. A local anesthetic blocks sensation only in the area of the pain, causing numbness. A dentist may give an injection of a local anesthetic such as novocaine to block pain before pulling a tooth or filling a cavity. A general anesthetic abolishes all sensation by rendering the patient unconscious.

Local Anesthetics

The first known local anesthetic drug was cocaine, a substance derived from the leaf of the coca plant. However, synthetic cocainelike drugs have since been developed to use in place of cocaine. These synthetics, such as novocaine, lidocaine, and benzocaine, last longer and avoid some of cocaine's undesirable side effects. For instance, they are less irritating to the heart and are not addictive. Although cocaine is non-narcotic, it is powerfully addicting for reasons not yet fully understood by scientists.

Local anesthetics fight pain by blocking nerve cells from producing the chemicals needed to send messages to the brain. Local anesthetics can also be injected into the area around the spinal cord to block the sending of pain messages to the brain. Called *epidural anesthesia*, this is used during some surgeries and during childbirth, when it is necessary to numb large areas yet keep the patient awake.

Some local anesthetics are available in over-the-counter products. For instance, sprays containing benzocaine are used to relieve the pain of sunburn, minor burns, cuts, scrapes, and other minor injuries. Although safe for most people when used as directed, these remedies should be used only on minor damage. A severe sunburn, particularly in a small child, or a large cut or burn should be seen by a doctor. Any injury that is likely to be infected, such as a bite from an animal or human, or a wound embedded with dirt or a foreign object, also warrants a doctor's attention. No over-the-counter remedy should be used by a person who is allergic to any of its ingredients. For that reason, allergy sufferers should always read the label and check with the pharmacist before taking an over-the-counter pain remedy.

General Anesthetics

There are two main types of general anesthetics: those that are inhaled as gases, such as halothane, *cyclopropane*, and nitrous oxide, and those that are injected, such as *sodium pentothal*. The inhaled general anesthetics, mixed with oxygen and administered through a mask, are used when it is necessary to keep a patient unconscious over a prolonged period, such as during major surgery.

Molecules of the inhaled gas travel through the lungs into the bloodstream, which carries them to the brain, where they take effect. When the patient wakes up, the side effects of inhaled general anesthetics may include grogginess, nausea, and congestion in the lungs, but these effects can be controlled with other medications. In any case, these side effects are a small price to pay for many lifesaving operations, such as heart surgery, which would be impossible without general anesthetics.

Injected general anesthetics, fed through an intravenous tube into a vein, are also carried to the brain. Compared to gaseous anesthetics, the side effects of injected anesthetics are less intense, fewer, and shorter in duration. Their most common side effect is grogginess. However, these anesthetics do not last as long as the gases—their molecules are quickly removed from the bloodstream by the liver—and the unconscious state they produce is not as deep, so they are more suitable for short procedures, such as tooth extraction and minor surgery.

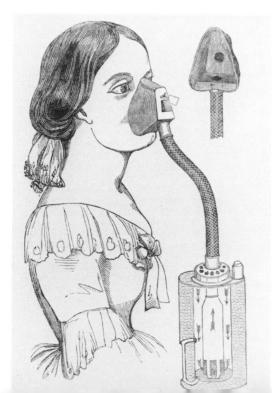

This 19th-century device offered a simple way to administer an inhaled gas. General anesthetics, which numb almost all bodily sensations, are typically used before and after surgery. Inhaled as a gas or administered by injection, they often induce unconsciousness.

General anesthetics are not available as over-the-counter drugs, and may only be administered by doctors. This is because individuals who are given general anesthesia need careful monitoring by medical professionals to make sure breathing and heart action remain normal while the patient is unconscious and as he or she awakens. Possible dangers may include asphyxia (lack of oxygen), liver toxicity (poisoning), or seizure activity.

TREATING THE CAUSE

A few drugs that relieve pain are not real pain-relieving drugs; neither analgesics nor anesthetics. They work by relieving the cause of pain— the condition that originally triggers pain messages—rather than blocking the pain itself. One example is the heart drug *nitroglycerin*, which is used against chest pain caused by coronary (heart) artery blockage. When *arteries*, blood vessels that supply oxygen to the heart, become partly blocked with fatty deposits, the heart receives less oxygen-bearing blood. If the vessels constrict even more due to anxiety or some other stress, or if the heart's need for oxygen increases due to exercise, the oxygen shortage can become critical, and the heart signals distress by sending pain messages to the brain.

Nitroglycerin has no effect on the pain messages themselves or on the brain. Instead, it acts to relax the coronary arteries so more oxygen-carrying blood can reach the heart. Once the heart begins receiving the increased oxygen supply, it stops sending distress signals and the chest pains ease. This does not cure the underlying heart-vessel blockage, but it does relieve the critical oxygen shortage.

In general, pain-relieving drugs work best against short-term pains caused by short-term conditions. For instance, the pain a person feels after having a tooth pulled arises from a condition that will heal. When it does, there will be no more pain, and no more need for pain relief. If the pain is mild, two aspirin tablets will probably relieve it. If a pain is more severe, a mild narcotic such as codeine may be prescribed. In either case, the drug will probably be taken in small amounts and for a short time, so there is little likelihood of serious side effects or addiction.

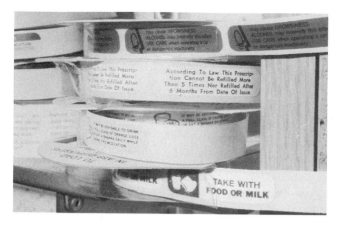

Although drugs provide hope for pain relief, they must be carefully monitored. When a person uses a drug for a prolonged period, he or she may need increasingly larger amounts to get the same degree of potency, a condition that can result in addiction.

CHRONIC PAIN RELIEF

Long-term or chronic pain presents a different problem. Pain, such as that caused by nerve damage, permanent injury, or serious illness, is likely to be more severe and require larger doses of a powerful pain reliever like morphine or one of the synthetic narcotics. Because the source of chronic pain does not heal, the pain does not go away; instead, it may last for weeks, months, or years, requiring the drug's use over a long period of time. The drug's pain-relieving effects are likely to diminish, as all narcotics become less effective over time. More and more of the drug will need to be taken to get the same relief; eventually, the drug may not work at all. At the same time, these potent drugs taken in large amounts are more likely to produce side effects, especially when taken for a long time. A person who continues taking a narcotic drug for an extended period also runs the risk of becoming addicted.

For all of these reasons, drugs are not a simple solution for the treatment of long-term pain. Through careful use of medication, however, doctors can minimize side effects and addiction while giving patients the most relief. But for long-term chronic pain, drugs are not the entire answer. Instead, a medically supervised program of pain-relieving medicines combined with nondrug pain management may produce more comfort, fewer side effects, and a better quality of life for the patient. The next chapter examines some of these very remarkable and useful nondrug methods of pain relief. Chapter 8 describes pain clinics, which offer in-depth treatment for chronic sufferers.

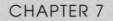

CHAPTER 7

PAIN RELIEF WITHOUT DRUGS

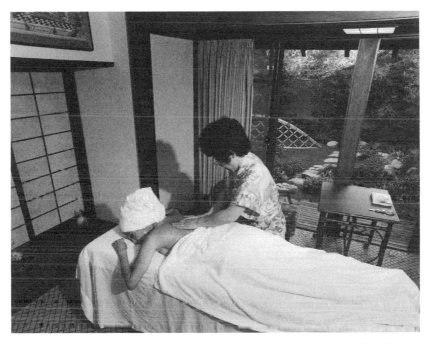

Massage is a common, uncomplicated method for pain relief. The vigorous rubbing performed by trained professionals is thought to block pain by overloading the body's pain-sending system.

Using drug-free methods of pain relief can be beneficial for several reasons. Most of these techniques can be done anywhere, need no special equipment, and have none of the undesirable effects of drugs. Often, combining several of the methods provides even more relief than using one alone.

EXTERNAL METHODS

Massage

One pain-control method that requires no drugs and no complicated equipment is massage. Most people perform simple massage on every-day bumps and bruises without even thinking about it, rubbing minor injuries to ease the pain. Many individuals receive massage from trained professionals, called *massage practitioners*, who press and rub the skin, muscles, and tendons to relieve tension and aches.

Massage therapy is thought to work because the nervous system can only send so many messages at one time. When vigorous rubbing overloads the system, the pain messages cannot get through. Because it can be somewhat painful, vigorous, deep massage may also stimulate the brain to release endorphins and other stop-pain chemicals. This explains why the good feeling of massage may last long after the actual rubbing has stopped.

Manipulation

Manipulation is the term used by chiropractors and other practitioners to describe the stretching, pulling, and twisting performed on the spine in order to relieve pain. The theory behind these manipulations is that pain is caused by spinal bones that have shifted out of alignment. Many physicians believe that no evidence has been shown to support this theory and that chiropractic treatment does not work for everyone. Nonetheless, many people believe that the technique has successfully relieved their pain. However, anyone suffering from pain that does not go away should be certain to visit a physician before continuing chiropractic treatment.

Heat

Applying heat to a painful area also overloads the transmitting system. For instance, putting a heating pad or hot water bottle against an aching back will often relieve the pain, at least temporarily. Physical therapists and other trained health technicians apply deep heat to painful areas by *diathermy*, electronic heating of deep areas of the muscles, bones, joints, and tendons, and by *ultrasound*, a method of producing heat by a concentrated application of ultrahigh-frequency sound waves. Regardless of how they are applied, the heat sensations are perceived by the brain while the pain signals are blocked because the nerves are busy sending the alternate messages. Heat treatment may also work by increasing blood flow to the injured area, causing pain chemicals such as bradykinin and prostaglandins to be washed out of the painful area.

Diathermy and ultrasound should be used only by trained medical professionals. Localized methods like heating pads and hot water bottles should be used with care to avoid burning the skin. They should not be used on infants or small children, people who have diabetes or other ailments that affect the circulation, or people who cannot feel the heat or communicate discomfort if their skin becomes too hot.

Cold

Anyone who has applied an ice pack to an aching area knows that cold can stop pain. Lowering the temperature reduces blood flow to the area, numbing the spot. A little-known fact is that ice applied to one part of the body can reduce pain in another part. In one study led by Dr. Ronald Melzack, toothache sufferers who received ice massage to the backs of their hands reported that tooth pain was relieved by at least 50%. Apparently, sensations produced by the ice blocked pain messages; the nervous system was so busy sensing the ice massage that it did not pay attention to pain messages from the aching teeth. Ice or cold for pain relief should be used with care because freezing the skin can cause injury.

Electrical Currents

The transcutaneous nerve stimulator is an electronic device that sends a tiny electrical current through nerves at the site of pain. Wired with electrodes taped to the skin, the current is not painful in itself, but works

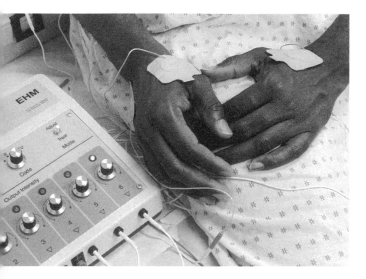

Another electronic technique is called TENS, or transcutaneous electrical nerve stimulation. It involves a device that sends electrical currents through electrodes taped to the skin near the nerves at an injured site.

by crowding out pain messages that would otherwise be transmitted to the brain. The technique, called transcutaneous electrical nerve stimulation or TENS for short, is convenient, safe for most people to use, and reasonably effective. However, TENS devices should be used only upon the recommendation of a physician, especially if an individual has a pacemaker.

According to Dr. Richard A. Sternbach, director of the Pain Treatment Center at the Scripps Clinic and Research Foundation and author of the book *Mastering Pain*, when TENS is used as part of a comprehensive pain management program it is effective in about 65% to 70% of patients. However, after a year of use, only about 50% of patients report continuing pain relief. Yet for those who do get long-term relief, the device is a simple solution to a serious problem.

INTERNAL TECHNIQUES

Surgery

"Acceptable long-term control of [chronic] pain is rarely achieved by surgery," say pain experts Ronald Melzack and Patrick D. Wall in their book *The Challenge of Pain*. Cutting pain-transmission nerves, in fact, disrupts the patterns of sensory messages received by the brain and may result in more pain for the patient than before.

Acupuncture

Acupuncture is a pain relief technique that has been practiced in China for more than 2,000 years. The technique relieves pain by inserting tiny needles into specific areas of the body, called *meridians*. In recent times, some scientists have suggested that it helps pain only by the placebo effect—it works simply because people believe it will. Yet studies have shown that acupuncture relieves pain in monkeys and mice as well as in people. Some scientists now think that, like many other nondrug methods of pain relief, acupuncture relieves discomfort by flooding the nerves with nonpainful but intense sensations, crowding out the pain messages with more numerous and intense messages.

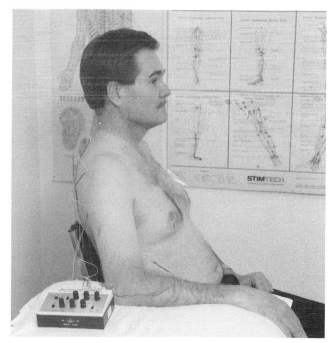

Acupuncture specialists relieve pain by inserting needles into designated points under the skin. The technique, practiced in China for thousands of years, has recently been updated, using an electronic device to rotate the needles after they have been inserted.

Acupuncture should be performed only by trained specialists whose needles are known to be absolutely clean, in order to avoid risk of infection with hepatitis or other serious viruses, such as AIDS.

MENTAL TECHNIQUES

Biofeedback

In the 1960s, a new technique was devised to help people gain voluntary control over body functions thought to be beyond their conscious influence—heart rate, blood pressure, muscle tension, and even brain waves. Electronic equipment was developed that could feed signals

Dr. Alvin Lake, director of biofeedback and psychological services at the Michigan Headache Clinic, oversees a patient undergoing biofeedback. The technique uses monitors to show the patient which mental states produce a desired physical result.

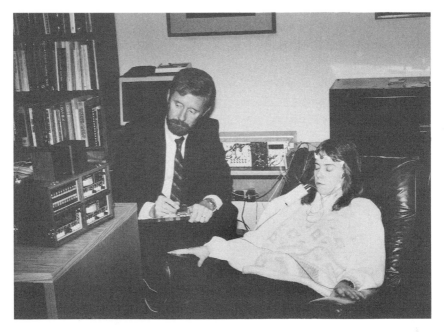

from these biological functions back to a monitor, so a person could see them and learn to control them mentally. Thus, the term *biofeedback* was coined.

It now appears that biofeedback can help control pain. For example, headaches caused by abnormally widened blood vessels in the brain may in fact be eased when the patient gains a certain amount of conscious control over the vessels. Generally, 75% of severe chronic headache sufferers eventually report getting some help from biofeedback.

However, additional studies showed that techniques that relax the individual and/or distract his or her attention from pain worked just as well as the complex techniques and expensive equipment needed for biofeedback control. Nevertheless, learning to gain some control over their body often helps patients relax more easily, which in turn helps to relieve pain. Additionally, patients find biofeedback so interesting that it gives a pain sufferer something to think about. This distraction also helps to reduce the perception of pain.

Hypnosis

Hypnosis is a technique that induces a trance state, a kind of awareness in which one is highly susceptible to suggestion. A person who is hypnotized or who learns self-hypnosis can accept useful suggestions, unless they go against his or her moral beliefs or desires. For instance, hypnosis may help a person quit smoking cigarettes but will not make him or her commit a crime. Some pain sufferers, by practicing self-hypnosis, can suggest to themselves that their pain is disappearing— and actually feel an improvement, although scientists do not fully understand why.

According to Sternbach, only about 10% of pain sufferers can learn to do hypnosis well enough to get meaningful pain relief, but the technique is so safe that many people find it worth trying. For the 1 in 10 who can truly banish pain this way, it improves life tremendously without drugs, side effects, or other undesirable results. Hypnosis or self-hypnosis should be used or taught only by trained, licensed specialists.

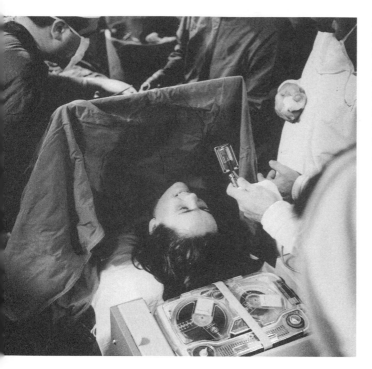

Hypnosis can be used to relieve pain during surgery without causing unconsciousness or side effects. Here, hypnotized patient Pierina Menegazzo, 19, smiled while having her appendix removed in Milan, Italy, in 1961.

Relaxation

Many people view relaxation as an activity to pursue for fun: playing a game, watching TV or a movie, listening to music, or hanging out with friends. Yet even when people think they are relaxing in these ways, their muscles may still be tense, with their necks or shoulders tight, their teeth and fists clenched. True relaxation produces a pleasant state of well-being, wherein the muscles are not tense, allowing the body to use its energy for healing, restorative, and disease-preventing abilities.

For most people, true bodily relaxation is not something that occurs by itself: People must deliberately create it, which sometimes means they must learn how to relax the body. This is especially true for individuals suffering from pain that, in turn, continually makes them tense. Pain feels worse when people are tense, so learning to relax the body through specific exercises is an important technique for relief.

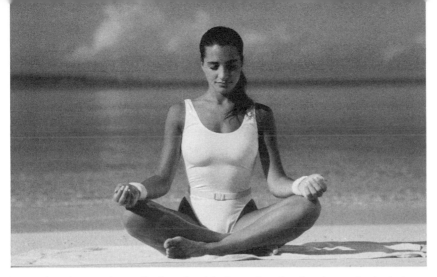

Yoga is a type of meditation that helps relax the body and mind. An even simpler method is transcendental meditation (TM), which can be practiced while sitting comfortably in a chair.

Two types of relaxation methods are *transcendental meditation* (TM) and *autogenic training.* Widely popular throughout the United States, TM involves sitting comfortably in a chair and repeating a mantra (a single, usually meaningless word) for 20 minutes. Autogenic training uses silent concentration on a specific command, such as "My heartbeat is calm and regular," to relax the body. A number of books, including Sternbach's *Mastering Pain,* describe relaxation exercises.

Exercise

Exercise is gaining recognition as a way to relieve some pains once thought to require major surgery. A 1980 study by surgeon Hubert Rosomoff at the University of Miami Comprehensive Pain and Rehabilitation Center showed that 86% of patients who were originally thought to need surgery for back pain could get better results—with fewer risks, less expense, and no surgical recovery period—from a program of muscle-strengthening exercises. The 7-year study of 7,000 patients concluded that much of the moderate to severe back pain people suffer does not come from damaged spinal bones or nerve injuries. Rather, this pain, which is bad enough in some cases to keep people out of work or school or to confine them to bed, comes from weak, out-of-shape muscles that could be strengthened and made less painful through exercise.

Other studies show that lack of exercise in a painful body part tends to make pain worse by disrupting the normal sensory messages the brain expects from that area. Unless a physician says that exercise will cause damage, staying active even when one has pain is a good idea. However, if continued exercise appears to create or worsen a pain, the individual should seek a doctor's opinion.

For severe or chronic pains, nondrug pain relief methods can be combined with other therapies in a program designed by specialists to take advantage of all the types of help modern medical science can offer.

CHAPTER 8

PAIN CLINICS

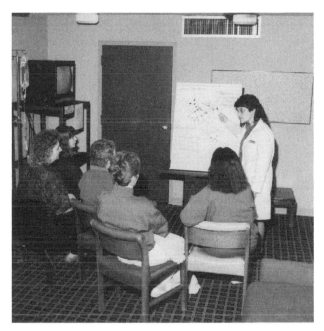

At the Michigan Headache Clinic, head nurse Elaine Yoglic teaches patients about the mechanisms that produce pain. Pain clinic staffs try to understand and explain causes of as well as cures for physical discomfort.

Dr. John Bonica, now the director emeritus of the Multidisciplinary Pain Center at the University of Washington School of Medicine, is known as the father of modern pain control. Bonica pioneered the idea that pain is influenced not only by physical causes, many of which are still not well understood, but also by mental, emotional, and social factors. He suggested that a person with chronic pain may need treatment by several medical specialists as well as by a range of other professionals, such as psychologists or psychiatrists, physical therapists, and social workers. In short, Bonica recognized that each person's pain problem is individual and complex and that a team effort is the most effective way to treat chronic pain.

In recent years, a number of pain clinics have developed around this idea. A person with chronic pain often visits doctor after doctor, searching for one who can provide relief, but finding no success. Each physician does his or her best, but the problem of chronic pain is often too difficult for one professional to solve alone. However, a patient who has been referred to a pain clinic by his or her family doctor or who decides independently to visit one gains access to a group of specialists who have up-to-date knowledge and specific training in treating chronic pain problems.

PREPARATION

A patient who begins treatment at a pain clinic often has a long history of pain and sometimes other physical problems. He or she may also have mental and emotional problems caused by suffering over an

A pain diary is an important component of treatment at a pain clinic. This patient is keeping a record of the frequency and intensity of her headaches; the diary will help doctors measure the ongoing effects of drugs and other treatments.

extended time period. The person's medical history is sent to the clinic, including records of illnesses and injuries, medical and surgical treatments, and the results of X rays and other tests. This medical record is usually examined by a doctor at the pain clinic before the patient's first appointment.

On the patient's first visit to the clinic, he or she meets the physician in charge of the case. The doctor talks with the person to learn not only about his or her pain but also about the individual's life as a whole and how the pain has affected it. A complete physical examination is also performed. Then, interacting with a team of specialists, the patient describes every detail of the pain, such as how it feels, how often it occurs, and where it hurts. The patient explains what brings on the pain, his or her past attempts at pain relief, and whether or not these were successful. The patient also lists any medications and pain remedies he or she is taking.

Information is also gathered about the pain sufferer's mental state—his or her beliefs, attitudes, and stresses. Psychologists may administer a personality test. The patient's feelings about the pain, and about what life would be like if it went away, are explored in depth. All of this information helps the staff at the pain clinic treat the patient as a unique individual with a specific problem, not just someone with another headache or another backache.

Finally, depending on the kind of pain the patient suffers, a variety of specialized tests may be performed. An *electromyograph*, for ex-

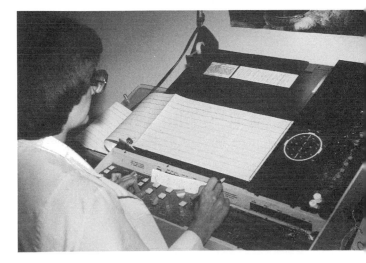

A technician at the Michigan Headache Clinic monitors EEG (electroencephalogram) tracings, which record the frequency of a patient's autonomic functions, including brain waves, heartbeat, breathing rate, and muscle activity.

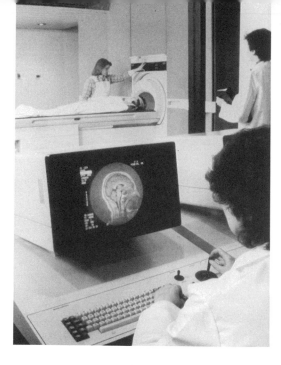

A magnetic resonance imaging (MRI) device produces a three-dimensional image of an area inside the body to help detect various disorders, such as blood clots and tumors. This procedure helps doctors treat the causes of pain as well as the symptoms.

ample, uses special sensors taped to the skin to measure muscle activity. It charts how the muscles function differently when the patient does or does not have pain. Another frequently performed test, especially for patients with headaches, is the *electroencephalogram* (EEG), which utilizes sensors taped to the patient's head to measure electrical activity in the brain. Knowing the patient's brain wave pattern is important in investigating headaches and other pains that may be coming from nervous system disorders.

If the clinic's team suspects that the patient's pain may be coming from a tumor, a blood clot, or an abnormality in the brain, a *computerized axial tomography* (CT) *scan* may be ordered. This produces a three-dimensional view of the inside of the body rather than the flat view provided by an X ray.

TREATMENT

When all the necessary information has been gathered, the members of the pain clinic team meet to discuss all that has been learned and to devise a treatment plan. The goal of the plan is to reduce the pain's frequency and severity and to lessen the need for painkilling drugs as

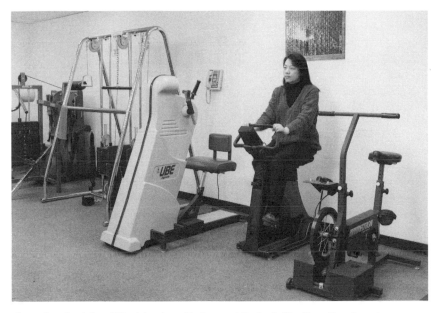

A patient at the Washington Pain and Rehabilitation Center demonstrates one aspect of treatment—exercise. Another room in the clinic contains different types of work stations that enable patients to learn proper posture to avoid pain on the job.

much as possible. The specialists also seek to help the patient live as normally as possible—to go to work or school, have friends, and pursue the daily activities he or she wants to without being crippled by pain. If drugs are needed, a medication program is designed to give the most relief possible with the fewest side effects.

The plan is different for every patient, but it may include better nutrition, an exercise program, different sleep patterns, and other life-style changes. Some patients may receive psychological help for the emotional problems their pain has brought on. Some may learn biofeedback, whereas others receive relaxation therapy or other pain relief methods that do not involve drugs.

Aside from the help it offers patients, another benefit of the pain clinic is that the variety of specialists who work together on the problem of pain are able to develop new pain therapies. Because the clinic's professionals keep careful records of what treatments have worked on

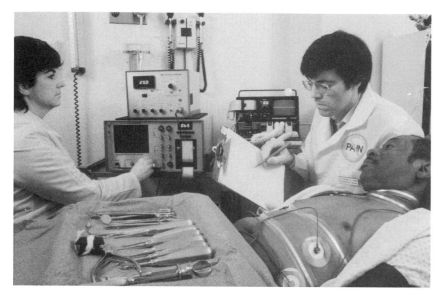

Researchers at the NIH Pain Research Clinic measure a patient's physical and psychological reactions to an intravenous drug administered before surgery. Specialists at pain clinics typically combine their different types of expertise to devise more specialized treatments.

various kinds of pain, they can use this information to treat new cases referred to the center.

Pain clinics can be expensive. Initial visits plus tests may total $700 or more, some of which may be covered by health insurance. Yet some patients say the results can be dramatic. For instance, pain clinics specializing in chronic headache pain report that 90% of their patients either improve dramatically or recover completely. Although not all pain responds this well to treatment, the help and research available at pain clinics may offer comfort and new prospects for the future.

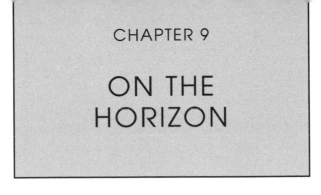

CHAPTER 9

ON THE HORIZON

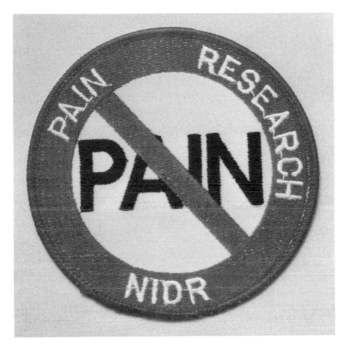

The National Institute of Dental Research (NIDR) uses a simple symbol to illustrate its attitude toward pain. The NIDR has greatly advanced the available research on how the body's hormones change in response to surgical stress.

Science has made stunning progress in the search for better and safer methods of pain relief. Still, some types of pain, such as the chronic pain caused by some types of cancer, cannot be relieved completely. There is also a need for more effective pain-relieving drugs that produce minimal side effects. Moreover, pain itself is not yet fully understood; researchers still have more to learn about the nervous system and about the way pain is sensed, transmitted, and perceived.

91

THE GATE CONTROL THEORY

A relatively new idea about how pain occurs is called the *gate control theory*. Developed in the 1960s by pain scientists Ronald Melzack, psychologist and research director of the Pain Center at Montreal General Hospital, and Patrick D. Wall, professor of anatomy at University College in London, the theory suggests that an area of the spinal cord called the *dorsal horn* contains specialized nerve cells that screen sensory messages traveling toward the brain. These nerve cells act as a gate that opens to allow painful sensations to reach the brain. Whether or not it opens depends on the strength and nature of the pain signal, compared to other messages traveling to and from the brain along the cord at the same time.

A slight pain signal plus an added message of anxiety may be enough to open the gate, whereas the pain message alone might not trigger the gate. One example is an injection: The event in itself is not dangerous and the pain alone is slight, but anxiety about illness or a fear of doctors, combined with memories of other, more painful medical procedures, may result in intense pain at the needle's prick.

In contrast, even a major pain message might not open the dorsal horn's gate cells if the nervous system is busy sending urgent messages about something else. For instance, a football player might not feel much pain during an exciting game even when a bone is broken. But later, when the game's excitement fades, the pain sets in. The gate, no longer busy with other nervous system messages, lets the pain messages through to the brain—with uncomfortable results.

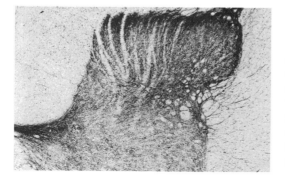

This micrograph illustrates a cross section of a dorsal horn in the spinal cord. This mechanism receives pain signals from nerves and transmits them to the brain. It is thought to determine which sensations reach the brain.

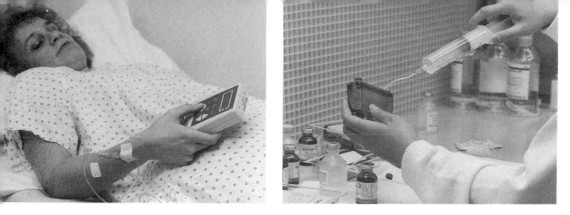

The Patient Controlled Analgesia (PCA) pump is one of the newer inventions for pain relief. Prefilled with the appropriate analgesic, a patient chooses when to self-administer the drug, and the quantity is regulated by a computer inside the pump.

The gate control theory also suggests that pain sensations can be changed by the actual pattern of messages traveling both to and from the brain. Thus, even the absence of messages can be perceived as pain in cases such as phantom pain, which occurs when an arm or leg that has been amputated still presents real pain to the brain. According to the theory, the disruption in the normal pattern of nerve messages from the absent leg is somehow perceived as painful. Scientists do not yet understand how this occurs.

Melzack and Wall, along with many other pain researchers, are working to learn more about the specific nerve-cell structures that are active in pain-inducing events. They are also investigating and identifying how various pain chemicals are made and how they function in the system. Another mystery that remains to be solved is the way in which the nervous system itself is controlled. When more is known about these functions, pain itself will be better understood and more controllable.

NEW SUBSTANCES

Meanwhile, efforts are underway to create new and safer drugs that will block the pain-producing effects of some of the body's own pain chemicals, while avoiding side effects such as addiction, drowsiness, risk of overdose, and long-term tolerance. Researchers use computers to model the narcotics' chemical structure and then change parts of the substances' chemical makeup to try to eliminate side effects.

One example is the development of an altered form of bradykinin by scientist Larry R. Steranka of Nova Pharmaceutical Corporation in Baltimore and Dr. Solomon H. Snyder of the Johns Hopkins University School of Medicine. This altered form binds to bradykinin receptors on nerve cells just as the normal chemical does, but it fails to stimulate a pain signal. In a sense, it jams the pain-sending mechanism. These bradykinin blockers are presently being tested in people against the painful symptoms of the common cold. The company also plans to test the substance in an ointment to treat the pain of burns.

For severe headache pain, the British company Glaxo Pharmaceuticals is testing a drug to raise the level of the stop-pain chemical serotonin in the brain. Dr. Seymour Solomon, director of the Headache Unit of Montefiore Medical Center in New York, says that 75% of patients in one group receiving the drug had partial or complete relief of headaches, with no, or mild, side effects. Another drug intended to prevent headaches is being tested by Eli Lilly and Company, an Indianapolis pharmaceutical manufacturer. Called *sergolexole maleate*, the drug seems to prevent blood vessels in the brain from widening abnormally, which keeps certain types of headaches from developing.

A substance called *capsaicin*, the active ingredient in hot peppers, is being studied for its pain-relieving effects. According to Dr. Paul Cotton in an article in the July 4, 1990, issue of the *Journal of the American Medical Association*, capsaicin causes a burning sensation when applied to the skin because it releases the pain chemical substance P from the tissues. However, it also stops more substance P from being made, so if the user endures the initial burning, all pain in the area is eventually reduced. The substance is being investigated for its usefulness against joint and muscle pain and to learn how it blocks substance P accumulation. Researchers are also examining the natural world of plants, animals, and minerals to find and test other substances that may contain pain-relieving properties.

SURGERIES

At present, surgery performed directly on the nerves, spinal cord, or brain has not produced effective results in relieving pain. Some cases

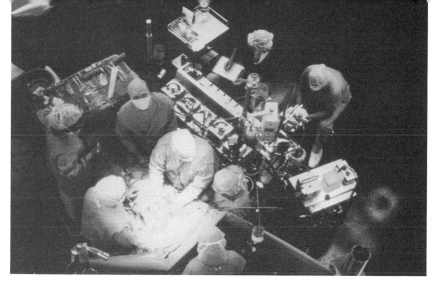

Unfortunately, most surgeries performed directly on the nerves, spinal cord, or brain have not proved successful. However, one recent technique uses an electronic brain implant to activate natural substances that block or kill pain signals within the brain.

of cluster headaches have been successfully treated through deadening a main nerve in the head, called the *trigeminal nerve*, by freezing it or injecting it with drugs. But the technique does not always work and usually causes one whole side of the face to be permanently numb and paralyzed.

A simpler method of cutting nerves to block the transmission of pain messages rarely works because pain messages do not usually travel along a single nerve. Rather, the signals seem to move through many nerves at once, similar to the way a wave flows through water. Scientists will need to learn more about the anatomy of nerves and the transmission of pain messages before similar, more reliable surgical techniques can be developed.

Transplantation

A special kind of nerve surgery, now being tested primarily on animals, may someday offer dramatic relief for many kinds of pain. George Pappas, head of the anatomy department at the University of Illinois, and colleague Jacqueline Sagan, a *neuropharmacologist* (a specialist in drugs that affect the nervous system), are studying the *chromaffin cells* of rats' adrenal glands, the glands that produce a wide variety of

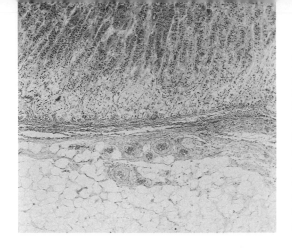

This cross section of an adrenal gland contains chromaffin cells, which produce large amounts of the body's natural pain relieving chemicals. Modern researchers are beginning to successfully graft these cells to different areas of the body to treat pain.

the body's chemicals (in humans as well as in rats). They are grafting the adrenal chromaffin cells into the spinal cords and brains of the rats. The transplanted cells make large amounts of enkephalins and norepinephrine.

The treated rats were so much less susceptible to pain and showed so few side effects that similar techniques are now being tried with humans. The results have led Dr. Pappas to predict that human adrenal-cell transplant surgery for pain relief may be common in as few as five years. Human adrenal chromaffin cell grafts to the spines of suffering cancer patients are now performed primarily for research, under the direction of cancer specialist Dr. Tapas DasGupta in Chicago.

In the meantime, another method of pain relief currently being studied utilizes an electronic brain implant that sends a tiny electric current into the brain. The device, which blocks pain messages and causes the release of natural painkilling substances in the brain, has been used at some medical centers, including the one at the University of Chicago. In one study described by pain researchers Melzack and Wall, 18 patients with severe pain received brain implants. The scientists reported that 12 subjects had partial pain relief, 1 had complete relief, and 5 had no relief. The technique remains under investigation to learn precisely how it works and whether it can be perfected to offer reliable pain relief to more patients.

No pain relief method is perfect. There is no magic pill or other therapy that will treat all types of pain. Yet as scientific advances are made, pain will become easier to control. Modern pain relief and treatments for ongoing pain are now safer, more accessible, and more effective than ever before.

APPENDIX:
FOR MORE INFORMATION

The following is a list of organizations that can provide further information about pain and related topics.

GENERAL INFORMATION

American Chronic Pain Association
P.O. Box 850
Rochlin, CA 95677
(916) 632-0922

International Pain Foundation
909 Northeast Forty-third Street,
    Suite 306
Seattle, WA 98105

National Chronic Pain Outreach
    Association, Inc.
7979 Old Georgetown Road, Suite 100
Bethesda, MD 20814-2429
(301) 652-4948

Pain Center
University of Alabama Medical Center
813 Sixth Avenue South
Birmingham, AL 35233
(205) 934-6174

ACUPUNCTURE

Acupuncture Foundation of Canada
57 Simcoe Street South, Suite 2M
Oshawa, Ontario L1H 7N1

Canada
(416) 723-8970

Acupuncture Research Institute
313 West Andrix Street
Monterey Park, CA 91754
(213) 722-7353

International College of Acupuncture and
    Electro-Therapeutics
(212) 781-6262

Traditional Acupuncture Institute
American City Building, Suite 100
Columbia, MD 21044
(301) 997-4888

BACK PAIN

Back Association of Canada
83 Cottingham Street
Toronto, Ontario M4V 1B9
Canada
(416) 967-4670

Canadian Chiropractic Association
1396 Eglinton Avenue West
Toronto, Ontario M6C 2E4
Canada
(416) 781-5656

North American Chronic Pain
   Association of Canada
c/o Dianne Cachie
6 Handel Court
Brampton, Ontario L6S 1Y4
Canada
(416) 793-5230

CANCER

American Cancer Society
1599 Clifton Road NE
Atlanta, GA 30329
(800) ACS-2345

Memorial Sloan-Kettering Cancer
   Center
1275 York Avenue
New York, NY 10021
(212) 639-2000

DRUG ABUSE

American Council for Drug Education
204 Monroe Street, Suite 100
Rockville, MD 20850
(301) 294-0600

Committees of Correspondence
57 Conant Street, Room 113
Danvers, MA 01923
(508) 774-2641

Do It Now Foundation
P.O. Box 25768
Tempe, AZ 85281
(602) 257-0797

Straight, Inc.
3001 Gandy Blvd.
St. Petersburg, FL 33702
(813) 576-8929

Target—Helping Students Cope with
   Alcohol and Drugs
P.O. Box 20626
11724 Plaza Circle

Kansas City, MO 64195
(816) 464-5400

HEADACHES AND MIGRAINES

Migraine Foundation
(416) 920-4916

National Headache Foundation
5252 North West Avenue
Chicago, IL 60625
(312) 878-7715
(800) 843-2256 (outside Illinois)
(800) 523-8858 (in Illinois)

HEART DISEASE

American Heart Association
7320 Greenville Avenue
Dallas, TX 75231
(214) 373-6300

The Coronary Club, Inc.
Cleveland Clinic Educational
   Foundation
9500 Euclid Avenue
Cleveland, OH 44195
(216) 444-3690

National Heart, Lung, and Blood
   Institute
National Institutes of Health
9000 Rockville Pike
Building 31, Room 4A21
Bethesda, MD 20892
(301) 496-4236

REYE'S SYNDROME

National Reye's Syndrome Foundation
426 North Lewis Street
Bryan, OH 43506
(419) 636-2679
(800) 233-7393 (outside Ohio)
(800) 231-7393 (in Ohio)

FURTHER READING

GENERAL INFORMATION

Aronoff, Gerald M., ed. *Evaluation and Treatment of Chronic Pain.* Baltimore: Urban & Schwarzenberg, 1985.

Bonica, John J., ed. *Pain.* New York: Raven Press, 1980.

Bresler, David E., and Richard Torubo. *Free Yourself from Pain.* New York: Simon & Schuster, 1979.

Cousins, Michael J., and Garry D. Phillips, eds. *Acute Pain Management.* New York. Churchill, 1985.

Epstein, Gloria J. *Help Yourself to Chronic Pain Relief: The Patient's Point of View.* Seattle: Manchester Group, 1981.

Fisk, James W. *Your Painful Neck and Back: A Complete Guide to Self-Help.* North Pomfret, VT: David & Charles, 1988.

Gelb, Harold. *Killing Pain Without Prescription.* New York: HarperCollins, 1980.

Kittredge, Mary. *Prescription and Over-the-Counter Drugs.* New York: Chelsea House, 1989.

Melzack, Ronald, and Patrick D. Wall. *The Challenge of Pain.* New York: Basic Books, 1983.

Smoller, Bruce, and Brian Schulman. *Pain Control: The Bethesda Program.* New York: Doubleday, 1982.

Sternbach, Richard A. *Mastering Pain.* New York: Ballantine Books, 1988.

Stimmel, Barry. *Pain, Analgesia, and Addiction: The Pharmacologic Treatment of Pain.* New York: Raven Press, 1983.

Tollison, C. David. *Managing Chronic Pain: A Patient's Guide.* New York: Sterling, 1982.

ACUPUNCTURE

Baxi, Nilesh, and C. H. Asrani. *Speaking of Alternative Medicine: Acupuncture, the Needle That Heals All Ailments.* New York: Apt Books, 1985.

Chailow, Leon. *The Acupunture Treatment of Pain: Safe and Effective Methods for Using Acupuncture in Pain Relief.* Scranton, PA: Inner Traditions International, 1984.

Lawson-Wood, Denis, and Joyce Lawson-Wood. *The Incredible Healing Needles: A Layman's Guide to Chinese Acupuncture.* York Beach, ME: Samuel Weiser, 1975.

Stievater, Eric H. *What Is Acupuncture? How Does It Work?* New York: State Mutual Books, 1980.

ANESTHESIA

Brown, Robert C. *Perchance to Dream: The Patient's Guide to Anesthesia.* Orlando, FL: Grune & Stratton, 1980.

Rupreht, J., et al., eds. *Anesthesia: Essays on Its History.* New York: Springer-Verlag, 1985.

BARBITURATES

Wesson, Donald R., and David E. Smith. *Barbiturates: Their Use, Misuse, and Abuse*. New York: Human Science Press, 1977.

HEADACHES AND MIGRAINES

Bassman, Stuart W., and William C. Wester II. *Hypnosis, Headache, and Pain Control: An Indirect Approach*. Columbus: Ohio Psychology, 1984.

Diamond, Seymour. *Coping with Your Headaches*. Madison, CT: International University Press, 1987.

Ehrmantraut, Harry C. *Headaches: The Drugless Way to Lasting Relief!* Berkeley, CA: Celestial Arts, 1987.

Mansfield, John. *The Migraine: The Drug-Free Solution*. Scranton, PA: Inner Traditions International, 1984.

Silverstein, Alvin, and Virginia B. Silverstein. *Headaches: All About Them*. New York: HarperCollins, 1984.

MASSAGE

Kellogg, J. H. *Art of Massage*. Watchung, NJ: Saifer, 1984.

Licht, Sidney, ed. *Massage, Manipulation, and Traction*. Melbourne, FL: Krieger, 1976.

Tappan, Frances. *Healing Massage Techniques: A Study of Eastern and Western Methods*. East Norwalk, CT: Appleton & Lange, 1978.

————. *Healing Massage Techniques: Holistic, Classic, and Emergency Methods*. East Norwalk, CT: Appleton & Lange, 1988.

NARCOTICS

Goldstein, Avram, ed. *The Opiate Narcotics: Neurochemical Mechanisms of Analgesia and Dependence.* Elmsford, NY: Pergamon Press, 1976.

Mule, S. J., and Henry Brill. *Chemical and Biological Aspects of Drug Dependence.* Boca Raton, FL: CRC Press, 1972.

Smith, J. E., and J. D. Lane. *Neurobiology of Opiate Reward Mechanisms.* New York: Elsevier Science, 1983.

THE NERVOUS SYSTEM

Chapouthier, G., and J. J. Matras. *The Nervous System and How It Functions.* Cambridge, MA: Abacus Press, 1986.

Essman, Walter B., ed. *Neurotransmitters, Receptors, and Drug Action.* Bridgeport, CT: Luce, 1980.

Kee, Leong S. *An Introduction to the Human Nervous System.* Athens: Ohio University Press, 1987.

GLOSSARY

acetaminophen a non-narcotic, synthetic drug similar to aspirin that is used for patients who are sensitive to aspirin; the active ingredient in Tylenol

acetylsalicylic acid a white crystalline solid derived from willow bark; the active ingredient in aspirin

acupuncture a technique developed by the Chinese to relieve pain by inserting fine needles at certain points

acute pain pain that is sharp, severe, and short-lived

adjuvant a drug added to another prescription drug to speed up or intensify its actions

afferent messages messages carried to the brain that deliver information about the body or the outside world

adrenaline a hormone that acts to avoid pain by raising blood pressure, which in turn raises blood sugar levels to provide the body with sudden energy and to stimulate the senses

amygdala a part of the limbic system that produces emotions in response to pain

analgesic a drug that relieves pain without causing loss of consciousness

anesthesia the loss of sensation resulting from the input of agents that block the passage of pain impulses to the brain

anesthetic a drug that relieves pain by producing numbness or unconsciousness

autogenic training a method of pain relief in which the patient concentrates on a specific command to relax his or her body

autonomic nervous system the part of the nervous system that controls the body's involuntary functions, such as breathing, digesting food, and pumping blood

axon the message-sending part of a nerve cell

barbiturate a class of addictive drugs that are generally used to reduce anxiety or induce euphoria; developed in 1903, barbiturates can be injected into the bloodstream to reduce anxiety before or after surgery

biofeedback a technique designed to teach individuals to control their autonomic nervous system; a monitoring device sounds a tone that enables the participant to reproduce the mental conditions that caused the desired change in pulse, blood pressure, brain waves, or muscle contractions

bradykinin a potent pain-producing chemical released when blood vessels are ruptured

causalgia pain with a burning sensation caused by damage to a peripheral nerve

central nervous system in vertebrates, the part of the body's nervous system containing the brain and the spinal cord

cerebral cortex the part of the brain that recognizes painful sensations and contains most of the brain's nerve cells

chronic pain pain that is ongoing or recurring

cluster headache a type of recurring vascular headache in which severe pain on one side of the head is often accompanied by sweating, tearing of the eyes, and blurred vision; occurs most frequently in cigarette smokers, especially male

computerized axial tomography scan (CT scan) a sectional, three-dimensional view of the inside of the body

dendrite the message-receiving part of a nerve cell

diathermy pain therapy in which a high-frequency current is used to heat muscles, bones, joints, and tendons

dorsal horn a section of the spinal cord containing specialized nerve cells that screen pain messages and regulate which ones travel to the brain

efferent messages instructions carried from the brain to the body

electromyograph an instrument that records the contractions of muscles; useful in graphing how the muscles function when the patient is or is not in pain

electroencephalogram (EEG) a recording of electrical activity in the brain; used to investigate headaches and other pains that may result from nervous system disorders

endorphins a group of proteins found in the brain that relieves pain

free endings nerve endings that fan out to gather information from outside the body through the skin

ganglion a group of nerve cells that is attached to and relays messages to the spinal cord

gate control theory a theory suggesting that nerve cells in the dorsal horn act as a gate to allow some painful sensations to reach the brain, depending on how their strength compares to other messages that may be attempting to reach the brain at the same time

hashish a narcotic extracted from the hemp plant that can be smoked or chewed to produce its euphoric effect

hippocampus a part of the limbic system that informs the cerebral cortex of new and unusual messages

hypothalamus a part of the brain responsible for autonomic regulatory functions such as breathing

ibuprofen an anti-inflammatory pain-relief drug used to treat arthritis; it is especially useful in patients with an intolerance to aspirin

interneurons nerve cells that act as "gatekeepers" to control the flow of pain messages between the synapses of the first and second nerve cells at an injured site

limbic system structures within the brain responsible for stimulating the cerebral cortex to notice new or unusual messages; it also affects the body's secondary responses and emotional reactions to such messages

massage manipulating, kneading, or applying pressure to the body to relieve tension

migraine headache a severe headache, recurring on one side of the head, that is often accompanied by nausea and vomiting

morphine an addictive narcotic drug used as an analgesic or sedative

motor nerves nerves that control muscle movement

muscle-contraction headache a tension headache; a dull, heavy, or pressing pain on both sides of the head and in the neck that may be due to a lack of serotonin, one of the brain's pain-regulating substances

narcotics drugs derived from the opium poppy that dull the senses and relieve pain

nerve blocking interrupting the passing of impulses through a nerve, using various types of anesthetics

neuralgia a type of chronic pain in which damaged nerves respond to sensations that are not ordinarily painful

neuron a nerve cell; a cell that can receive and transmit nervous impulses; contains an axon and dendrites

neuropharmacologist a specialist who deals with the action of drugs on and in the nervous system

neurotransmitters substances that carry nerve impulses across a synapse

nociception perception of pain or injury by the nerve endings

nociceptor a nerve ending that receives painful stimuli

non-narcotics nonaddictive analgesics that block pain but do not work on the central nervous system

opiate a pain relief drug derived from opium

opioids synthetic narcotics that perform opiatelike activities but which are not derived from opium

opium an addictive narcotic drug derived from certain poppy plants that relieves pain but that can also produce hallucinations and, in excessive dosages, result in coma or death

peripheral nervous system the part of the nervous system that registers physical sensations and carries information about them to and from the brain

phantom pain pain that occurs in a body part that no longer exists; after an arm or leg is amputated, the phantom pain may be felt, as if the limb were still there

pharmacology the study of drugs and their properties and reactions

premenstrual syndrome(PMS) a condition occurring in some women prior to menstruation; symptoms may include irritability, insomnia, fatigue, depression, headache, anxiety, and lower abdominal pain

psychogenic pain a pain that is not caused by a physical ailment but by severe depression or other emotional disorders

Reye's syndrome an often fatal disease of the brain marked by symptoms of fever, vomiting, swelling of the kidneys and brain, and fatty infiltration of the liver; can be linked to the ingestion of aspirin by children suffering from a viral infection

spinal cord the bundle of nerves running through the center of the spinal column that serves as a pathway for messages between the brain, the torso, and the limbs

substance P a chemical in the body that produces redness, heat, and swelling in the area of an injury in response to pain

sympathectomy the surgical removal of autonomic nerves to relieve causalgia

synapse the tiny gap between two nerves

transcendental meditation (TM) a meditation technique that involves the repetition of a mantra, or incantation; used to induce relaxation or relieve pain

transcutaneous electronic nerve stimulator (TENS) an electronic device that relieves pain by transmitting small electrical currents via needles inserted through the skin

trephining cutting pieces of bone from the skull with a sawlike instrument called a trephine; also an early type of brain surgery performed in South America in which the patient's skull was opened to release evil spirits believed to be causing pain

ultrasound a method of producing pain-relieving heat by applying high-frequency sound waves to a sensitive area

vascular headache a pounding or thudding pain that arises when the walls of blood vessels in the brain become dilated; can be caused by foods containing nitrites, monosodium glutamate (MSG), and caffeine

vasodilator a substance that causes blood vessels to widen

voluntary nervous system the part of the nervous system that controls voluntary activities such as walking and talking

INDEX

PICTURE CREDITS

Air Force Pathology Institute: p. 96; E. S. Beckwith/Taurus Photos: p. 74; Bettmann Archive: p. 18; © 1908 H. B. Conyers Collection, Library of Congress: cover; Eric B. Jones: pp. 23, 55, 56, 69 (left and right); Michael Keller/FPG International: p. 83; Photo by Michael Latil, courtesy of Washington Pain and Rehabilitation Center, Inc.: pp. 79, 89; Library of Congress: pp. 14, 46; Michigan Headache Clinic: pp. 80, 85, 86, 87; National Institute of Dental Research, National Library of Medicine: pp. 35, 38, 49, 90, 91, 92; National Institutes of Health: pp. 48, 51, 62, 65, 88, 95; National Library of Medicine: pp. 13, 15, 16, 17, 20, 41, 42, 53, 58, 60, 67, 72; Photo by Edward Owen, courtesy of Georgetown University Medical Center Pain Clinic: pp. 78, 93 (left and right); Original illustrations by Nisa Rauschenberg: pp. 24, 25, 27, 28, 29, 30, 32, 37, 43; Reuters/Bettmann Archive: p. 33; Charles Schneider/FPG International: p. 75; Smithsonian Institution: p. 21; United Nations: pp. 39, 52, 66; UPI/Bettmann Archive: pp. 45, 82

Mary Kittredge is the author of seven novels for adults and more than a dozen books on history, science, and health for young people, including *The Respiratory System, Prescription and Over-the-Counter Drugs,* and *The Human Body: An Overview* in the Chelsea House ENCYCLOPEDIA OF HEALTH. Educated at Trinity College in Hartford and at the University of California Medical School in San Francisco, she is certified as a respiratory care technician by the American Association for Respiratory Therapy and has been associate editor of the medical journal *Respiratory Care.* Her writing awards include the Ruel Crompton Tuttle Essay Prize and the Mystery Writers of America Robert L. Fish Award for best first short mystery fiction of 1986.

Dale C. Garell, M.D., is medical director of California Children Services, Department of Health Services, County of Los Angeles. He is also associate dean for curriculum at the University of Southern California School of Medicine and clinical professor in the Department of Pediatrics & Family Medicine at the University of Southern California School of Medicine. From 1963 to 1974, he was medical director of the Division of Adolescent Medicine at Children's Hospital in Los Angeles. Dr. Garell has served as president of the Society for Adolescent Medicine, chairman of the youth committee of the American Academy of Pediatrics, and as a forum member of the White House Conference on Children (1970) and White House Conference on Youth (1971). He has also been a member of the editorial board of the *American Journal of Diseases of Children.*

C. Everett Koop, M.D., Sc.D., is former Surgeon General, deputy assistant secretary for health, and director of the Office of International Health of the U.S. Public Health Service. A pediatric surgeon with an international reputation, he was previously surgeon-in-chief of Children's Hospital of Philadelphia and professor of pediatric surgery and pediatrics at the University of Pennsylvania. Dr. Koop is the author of more than 175 articles and books on the practice of medicine. He has served as surgery editor of the *Journal of Clinical Pediatrics* and editor-in-chief of the *Journal of Pediatric Surgery.* Dr. Koop has received nine honorary degrees and numerous other awards, including the Denis Brown Gold Medal of the British Association of Paediatric Surgeons, the William E. Ladd Gold Medal of the American Academy of Pediatrics, and the Copernicus Medal of the Surgical Society of Poland. He is a chevalier of the French Legion of Honor and a member of the Royal College of Surgeons, London.